About the NCCN Guidelines for Patients®

National Comprehensive Cancer Network®

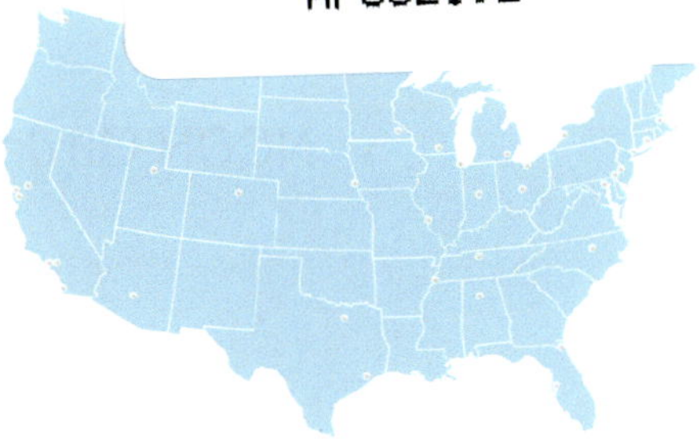

Did you know that top cancer centers across the United States work together to improve cancer care? This alliance of leading cancer centers is called the National Comprehensive Cancer Network® (NCCN®).

Cancer care is always changing. NCCN develops evidence-based cancer care recommendations used by health care providers worldwide. These frequently updated recommendations are the NCCN Clinical Practice Guidelines in Oncology (NCCN Guidelines®). The NCCN Guidelines for Patients plainly explain these expert recommendations for people with cancer and caregivers.

These NCCN Guidelines for Patients are based on the NCCN Clinical Practice Guidelines in Oncology (NCCN Guidelines®) for Acute Myeloid Leukemia, Version 2.2024 – March 22, 2024.

View the NCCN Guidelines for Patients free online
NCCN.org/patientguidelines

Find an NCCN Cancer Center near you
NCCN.org/cancercenters

Connect with us

Supporters

NCCN Guidelines for Patients are supported by funding from the NCCN Foundation®

NCCN Foundation gratefully acknowledges the following corporate supporters for helping to make available these NCCN Guidelines for Patients: AbbVie, Pfizer Inc., and Servier.

NCCN independently adapts, updates, and hosts the NCCN Guidelines for Patients. Our corporate supporters do not participate in the development of the NCCN Guidelines for Patients and are not responsible for the content and recommendations contained therein.

To make a gift or learn more, visit online or email

NCCNFoundation.org/donate

PatientGuidelines@NCCN.org

Contents

NCCN Foundation seeks to support the millions of patients and their families affected by a cancer diagnosis by funding and distributing NCCN Guidelines for Patients. NCCN Foundation is also committed to advancing cancer treatment by funding the nation's promising doctors at the center of innovation in cancer research. For more details and the full library of patient and caregiver resources, visit NCCN.org/patients.

National Comprehensive Cancer Network (NCCN) and NCCN Foundation
3025 Chemical Road, Suite 100, Plymouth Meeting, PA 19462 USA

1
AML basics

Acute myeloid leukemia (AML) is a type of blood cancer that starts in the stem cells of bone marrow. There are many subtypes of AML found in adults. This chapter will provide an overview of AML.

Blood

Acute myeloid leukemia (AML) is a type of blood cancer. Blood is a tissue. A tissue is a group of cells that work together to perform a function. Blood's function is to move oxygen and nutrients throughout the body and carry away waste. Blood also plays an important role for the immune system and in preventing bleeding.

Blood cells

Your blood contains different types of cells that float in plasma. Plasma is a clear, yellowish fluid made up of mostly water. More than half of your blood is plasma and the rest is made up of blood cells.

There are 3 types of blood cells:

- Red blood cells (erythrocytes)
- White blood cells (leukocytes), which include granulocytes (neutrophils), monocytes, lymphocytes, and others
- Platelets (thrombocytes)

Blood cells have important jobs. Red blood cells (RBCs) carry oxygen throughout the body. White blood cells (WBCs) fight infections. Platelets (PLTs) help control bleeding. Blood cells are being replaced in your body all the time. Many have a short lifespan. Some white blood cells live less than one day. Your body makes one million red blood cells every second!

Blood stem cells

Bone marrow contains stem cells. A blood stem cell is an immature cell that can develop into a red blood cell, white blood cell, or platelet.

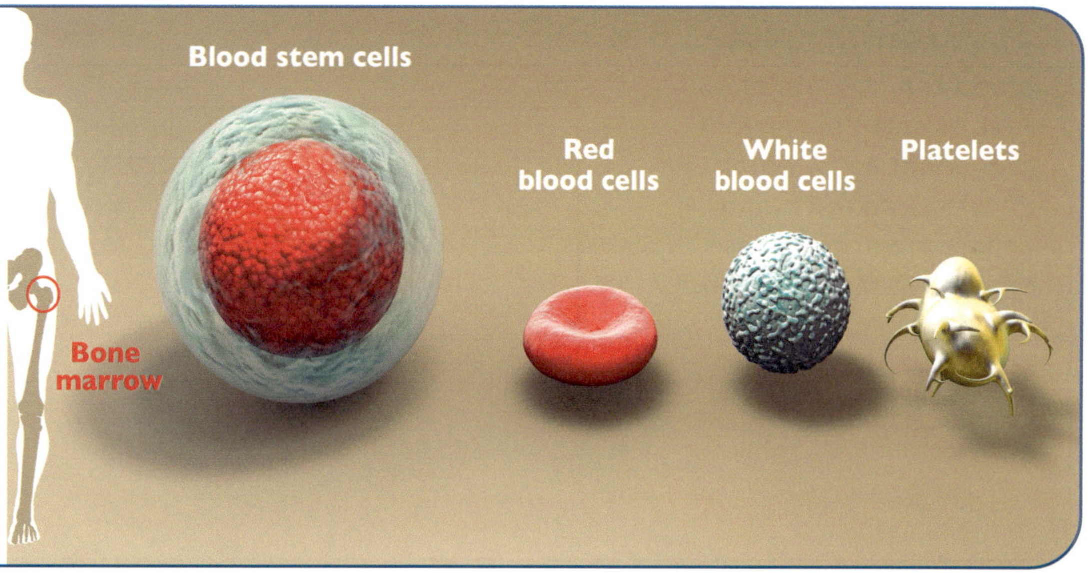

How blood cells are formed

Bone marrow is the organ that creates blood in our body. Bone marrow is the sponge-like tissue in the center of most bones. Inside your bone marrow are early blood-forming cells called blood (hematopoietic) stem cells. Stem cells multiply so we have enough supply for our lifetime. Some of those stem cells also gradually turn into blood cells. This process is called differentiation.

At any given time, bone marrow will have cells in various stages of development, from very immature to almost fully mature. After a blood stem cell develops into a red blood cell, white blood cell, or platelet, it is released in your bloodstream as needed.

AML starts in the blood stem cells and makes abnormal myeloblasts, also called blasts or leukemia cells.

Blasts

A blast is an immature white blood cell. Blasts are committed to becoming a type of blood cell. Lymphoblasts normally mature into lymphocytes, a type of white blood cell. Myeloblasts are responsible for all other non-lymphoid blood cells in bone marrow, such as granulocytes (another type of white blood cell).

Blood cell formation

All blood cells start as blood stem cells. A blood stem cell has to mature or go through many stages to become a red blood cell, white blood cell, or platelet. AML affects the myeloid progenitor cells, which develop into red blood cells, granulocytes (a type of white blood cell), and platelets.

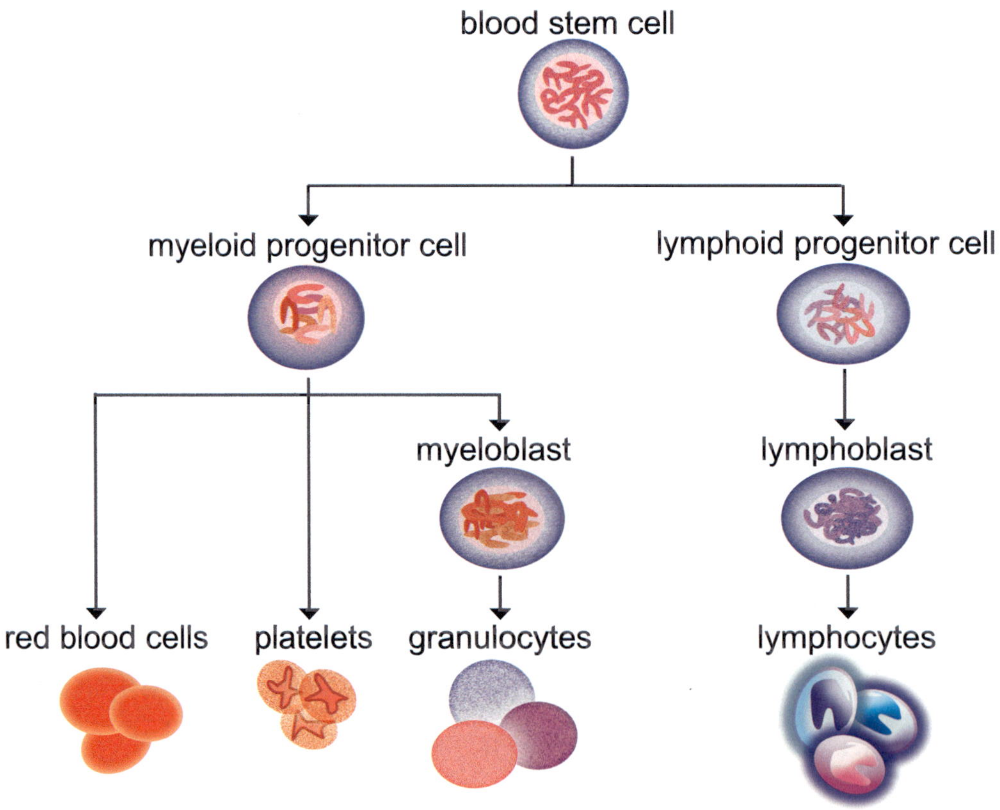

Acute myeloid leukemia

In acute myeloid leukemia (AML), changes stop myeloid blasts (or myeloblasts) from becoming mature blood cells. As a result, there is a buildup of blasts in the bone marrow and blood. In turn, there are not enough healthy red blood cells, platelets, and white blood cells. This causes serious health issues. For this reason, AML is fatal if left untreated.

Traditionally, to be diagnosed with AML, 20 percent (20%) or more myeloblasts must be present in the marrow or blood. This means that at least 1 out of every 5 marrow cells are blasts. However, myelodysplastic syndromes (MDS) can also have increased blasts. As a result, MDS with 10% to 19% blasts is called MDS/AML. In certain cases, a diagnosis of AML is possible with any number of blasts, particularly if certain gene mutations or abnormal chromosomes are also present.

Subtypes of AML

There are many subtypes of AML. They are grouped and treated based on the presence or absence of certain gene mutations or abnormal chromosomes and other factors.

Treatment chapters in this book are divided into:

- Acute myeloid leukemia (AML)
- Acute promyelocytic leukemia (APL)
- Blastic plasmacytoid dendritic cell neoplasm (BPDCN)

Key points

- AML starts in the blood stem cells and makes abnormal myeloblasts, also called blasts or leukemia cells.
- Changes stop myeloid blasts from becoming mature blood cells. As a result, there is a buildup of blasts in the bone marrow and blood making it hard for blood to do its work.
- A traditional diagnosis of AML requires that 20 percent (20%) or more myeloid blasts must be present in the bone marrow or blood. This means that at least 1 out of every 5 marrow cells are blasts.
- In certain cases, a diagnosis of AML is possible with any number of blasts, particularly if certain gene mutations or abnormal chromosomes are also present.
- There are many subtypes of AML. They are grouped and treated based on gene mutations and other factors.

2
Testing for AML

Accurate testing is needed to diagnose and treat acute myeloid leukemia (AML). This chapter presents an overview of possible tests you might receive and what to expect.

Test results

Accurate testing is needed to diagnose and treat AML. A diagnosis of AML is based on the presence of myeloid blasts in the bone marrow or blood. The number of blasts required to be diagnosed with AML can vary. Traditionally, the number of blasts must be 20 percent (20%) or more. This means that at least 1 out of every 5 marrow cells are blasts. However, a diagnosis of AML is possible with any number of blasts, particularly if certain gene mutations or abnormal chromosomes are also present.

Unlike other cancers of organs, like lung cancer or breast cancer, AML does not have stages. Instead, testing looks for specific gene mutations or abnormal chromosomes, which can tell your care team how aggressive your leukemia might be.

Results from blood tests, bone marrow aspirate and biopsy, and imaging studies will be used to guide your treatment plan. It is important you understand what these tests mean. Ask questions about your test results. Online patient portals are one way to access your test results. Please wait to discuss the results with your doctor or health care team.

Keep these things in mind:

- It's beneficial to have a support system in place during diagnosis and treatment. Enlist the help of friends, family members, or peers who can provide transportation, meals, and emotional support. These can be different people for different tasks or change over time.
- Consider bringing someone with you to doctor visits if possible, or have someone on the phone or join you for telehealth visits.
- Don't hesitate to ask questions and take notes during appointments. Write down questions and ask a friend or family member to take notes.
- Organize your medical documents, including insurance forms, medical records, and test results. Keep a list of contact information for your care team and update your primary care physician (PCP) regarding any changes. Include details about the specific type of cancer, treatment, and dates in your contact list.
- Set up a MyChart or health record account if it's available, which can help you track your appointments and communicate with your care team. Remember, in many places the MyChart or portal messages are not immediately seen by a nurse or physician, so ask your care team how best to communicate with them, especially in an emergency.

For possible tests and procedures, **see Guide 1.**

General health tests

Medical history

A medical history is a record of all health issues and treatments you have had in your life. Be prepared to list any illness or injury and when it happened. Bring a list of old and new medicines and any over-the-counter (OTC) medicines, herbals, or supplements you take. Some supplements interact and affect medicines that your care team may prescribe. Tell your care team about any symptoms you have. A medical history, sometimes called a health history, will help determine which treatment is best for you.

Family history

Some cancers and other diseases can run in families. Your doctor will ask about the health history of family members who are blood relatives. This information is called a family history. Ask family members on both sides of your family about their health issues like heart disease, cancer, and diabetes, and at what age they were diagnosed. It's important to know the specific type of cancer, or where the cancer started, and if it is in multiple locations. Those with a family history of leukemia, blood cancer or abnormalities, or certain genetic mutations might be referred to genetic counseling.

Guide 1 Possible tests and procedures: AML
Medical history and physical exam
Complete blood count (CBC), platelets, differential, comprehensive metabolic panel (CMP), uric acid, lactate dehydrogenase (LDH), B12, and folic acid
Blood clotting tests
Bone marrow aspirate and biopsy with AML biomarker and genetic testing
Human leukocyte antigen (HLA) typing
Brain CT without contrast, if central nervous system (CNS) bleed suspected
Brain MRI with contrast, if leukemic meningitis suspected
FDG-PET/CT, if leukemia outside the blood and bone marrow (extramedullary) suspected
Lumbar puncture (LP)
Heart tests

Physical exam

During a physical exam, your doctor may:

- Check your temperature, blood pressure, pulse, and breathing rate
- Check your height and weight
- Listen to your lungs and heart
- Look in your eyes, ears, nose, and throat
- Feel and apply pressure to parts of your body to see if organs are of normal size, are soft or hard, or cause pain when touched
- Feel for enlarged lymph nodes in your neck, underarm, and groin

Blood tests

Blood tests check for signs of disease and how well organs are working. They require a sample of your blood, which is removed through a needle placed into a vein. Be prepared to have many blood tests during AML treatment and recovery to check treatment results, blood counts, and the health of organs like your liver and kidneys.

Tests described next are listed alphabetically and not in order of importance.

B12 and folic acid

Vitamin B12 and folic acid (folate) work with vitamin C to help the body make new proteins. They are needed for normal red blood cell (RBC) and white blood cell (WBC) formation. B12 and folic acid levels will be monitored. You may be given vitamin supplements, if needed.

Blood clotting tests

Your body stops bleeding by turning blood into a gel-like form. The gel-like blood forms into a solid mass called a blood clot. Clotting is a process or series of events. Proteins, called coagulation factors, are needed for clotting. They are made by the liver. These tests are known together as a coagulation panel or disseminated intravascular coagulation (DIC) panel.

It is standard to screen for clotting problems. An impaired clotting process is common in leukemia. This is called coagulopathy. You may have bleeding and bruises.

Blood urea nitrogen

Blood urea nitrogen (BUN) is a waste product filtered out of the blood by the kidneys. A high level of BUN can be a sign your kidneys aren't working well.

Comprehensive metabolic panel

A comprehensive metabolic panel (CMP) is a test that measures 14 different substances in your blood. It is usually done on the plasma part of your blood. A CMP provides important information about how well your kidneys and liver are working, among other things.

Complete blood count and differential

A complete blood count (CBC) measures the levels of red blood cells (RBCs), white blood cells (WBCs), and platelets (PLTs) in your blood. A CBC is a key test that gives a picture of your overall health. AML often causes low counts of healthy blood cells, but it can also present with a high number of abnormal, malignant (abnormal) white blood cells.

There are several types of white blood cells. A differential counts the number of each type of white blood cell. It also checks if the counts are in balance with each other. This test may show a high number of blasts in the blood.

Your care team will pay particular attention to the following CBC measurements:

- Hemoglobin (Hgb) is a measurement of how much oxygen can move through blood and if a red blood cell transfusion might be needed.
- Platelets (PLT) are cells that make the clot, thus preventing or stopping the bleeding.
- Absolute neutrophils (ANC) are the cells that fight with bacteria and protect us from infections.
- Blasts or leukemia cells can sometimes be detected in the blood and usually are reported as a percentage of cells.

Creatinine

Creatinine is a waste produced in the muscles. Every person generates a fixed amount of creatinine every day based on how much muscle they have. It is filtered out of the blood by the kidneys. The level of creatinine in the blood tells how well the kidneys are working. Higher levels of creatinine mean the kidneys aren't working as well as they were when someone had lower levels of creatinine.

Electrolytes

Electrolytes help move nutrients into cells and help move waste out of cells. Electrolytes are ions or particles with electrical charges that help the nerves, muscles, heart, and brain work as they should. Your body needs electrolytes to function properly. Phosphate (PO4), a type of electrolyte, is important for strong bones and teeth. Too much phosphate in blood can be a sign your kidneys aren't working well.

Iron

Iron is important in maintaining body functions such as producing hemoglobin, the molecule in your blood that carries oxygen. You might be monitored for low levels of iron called iron deficiency. You may be given an intravenous (IV) iron supplement, if needed. It is possible to have too much iron in the body called overload. Therefore, only take what is prescribed by your doctor.

Lactate dehydrogenase

Lactate dehydrogenase (LDH) or lactic acid dehydrogenase is a protein found in most cells. Dying cells release LDH into blood. Fast-growing cells also release LDH. High levels of LDH can be a sign of AML.

Liver function tests

Liver function tests (LFTs) look at the health of your liver by measuring chemicals that are made or processed by the liver. Levels that are too high or low signal that the liver is not working well.

Phosphate

Cells have a lot of phosphate in them. Therefore, when many cells are breaking down at the same time, the levels of phosphate in the blood can go up. Your kidneys help get rid of extra phosphate, but too much phosphate in the blood can also damage the kidneys, making it harder to get the levels back down to normal.

Uric acid

Uric acid is released by cells when DNA breaks down. It is a normal waste product that dissolves in your blood and is filtered by the kidneys where it leaves the body as urine. Too much uric acid in the body is called hyperuricemia. With AML, it can be caused by a fast turnover of white blood cells. High uric acid might be a side effect of chemotherapy or radiation therapy. Very high levels of uric acid in the blood can damage the kidneys.

Be prepared to have many blood tests.

HLA typing

A human leukocyte antigen (HLA) is a protein found on the surface of most cells. It plays an important role in your body's immune response. HLAs are unique to each person. They mark your body's cells. Your body detects these markers to tell which cells are yours. In other words, all your cells have the same set of HLAs. Each person's set of HLAs is called the HLA type or tissue type.

HLA typing is a test that detects a person's HLA type. This test is done before a donor (allogeneic) blood stem cell transplant, also called a hematopoietic cell transplant (HCT). To find a donor match, your proteins will be compared to the donor's white blood cells to see how many proteins are the same. A very good match is needed for a transplant to be a treatment option. Otherwise, your body will reject the donor cells or the donor cells will react against your body. Blood samples from you and your blood relatives will be tested first.

Performance status

Performance status (PS) is a person's general level of fitness and ability to perform daily tasks. Your state of general health will be rated using a PS scale called Eastern Cooperative Oncology Group (ECOG). PS is one factor taken into consideration when choosing a treatment plan. Your preferences about treatment are always important.

The ECOG PS scores are as follows:

- **PS 0** means the person is fully active.
- **PS 1** means the person is still able to perform light to moderate activity, but with some limitations.
- **PS 2** means the person is limited to the chair or bed less than half of the time and still able to care for self.
- **PS 3** means the person is limited to the chair or bed more than half of the time.
- **PS 4** means the person is totally confined to the bed or chair and completely unable to care for self.

Good PS is usually PS 0 or PS 1.

Bone marrow tests

A diagnosis of AML is often confirmed using a bone marrow aspirate and bone marrow biopsy. Your bone marrow is like a sponge holding liquid and cells. An aspirate takes some of the liquid and cells out of the sponge, and a biopsy takes a piece of the sponge. A bone marrow aspirate and biopsy are often done at the same time.

Leukemia starts in the bone marrow. To diagnose AML, samples of bone marrow must be removed and tested before starting any treatment. Your sample should be reviewed by a pathologist who is an expert in the diagnosis of AML. This review is often referred to as histology, histopathology, or hematopathology review. The pathologist will note the overall appearance and the size, shape, and type of your cells.

A bone marrow aspirate and biopsy is a bedside procedure. It is not a surgery and does not require an operating room. Your care team will try to make you as comfortable as possible during the procedure. The samples are usually taken from the back of the hip bone (pelvis). You will likely lie on your belly or side. For an aspirate, a hollow needle will be pushed through your skin and into the bone. Liquid bone marrow will then be drawn into a syringe. For the biopsy, a wider needle will be used to remove a small piece of bone. You may feel bone pain at your hip for a few days. Your skin may bruise.

- If the blastic plasmacytoid dendritic cell neoplasm (BPDCN) subtype of AML is suspected, you might also have a lymph node biopsy or a skin lesion biopsy.

Flow cytometry

Flow cytometry (FCM) is a laboratory method used to detect, identify, and count specific cells. Flow cytometry involves adding a light-sensitive dye to cells. The dyed cells are passed through a beam of light in a machine. The machine measures the number of cells, things like the size and shape of the cells, and other unique features of cells.

A complete blood test can count the number of white blood cells, but it cannot detect the subtle differences between different types of blood cancers. Flow cytometry can detect these subtle differences. The most common use of flow cytometry is in the identification of markers on cells, particularly in the immune system (called immunophenotyping).

Immunophenotyping

Immunophenotyping is a process that uses antibodies to detect the presence or absence of white blood cell antigens called biomarkers. These antigens are proteins that can be found on the surface of or inside white blood cells. Certain biomarkers are targeted in AML treatment.

Immunohistochemistry

Immunohistochemistry (IHC) is a special staining process that involves adding a chemical marker to cells. The cells are then studied using a microscope. IHC looks for the immunophenotype of cells from a biopsy or tissue sample.

Bone marrow aspirate and biopsy

Samples of bone and marrow are removed in a biopsy.

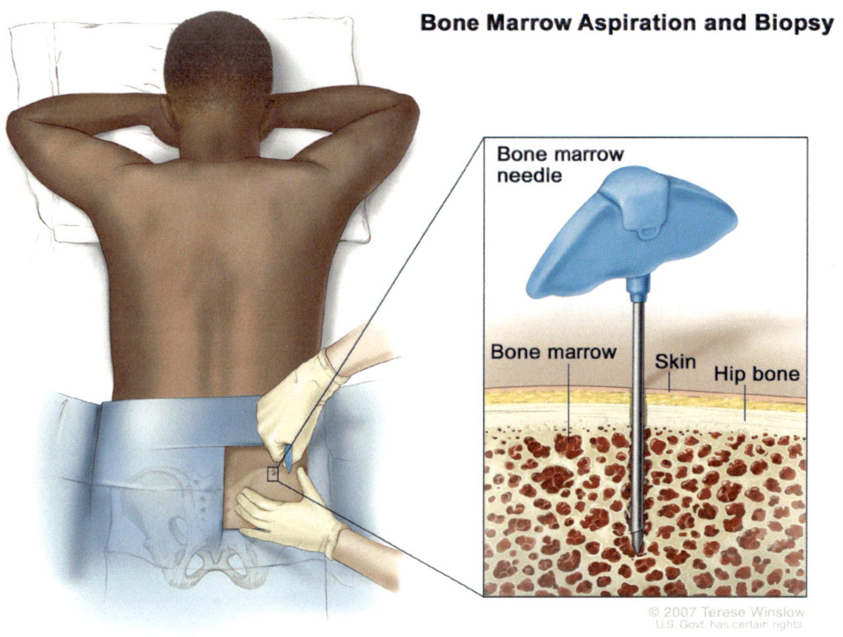

Testing for AML biomarkers and genetic changes

Biomarker testing includes tests of genes or their products (proteins) and identifies the presence or absence of mutations and certain proteins that might suggest the leukemia subtype. Genetic and biomarker tests are used to learn more about your type of AML, to target treatment, and to determine the likely path your cancer will take (prognosis). This genetic testing is different from family history genetic testing and genetic cancer risk testing. AML genetic testing looks for changes only in the leukemia cells that have developed over time, and not changes in the rest of your body's cells. It is sometimes called molecular testing, tumor profiling, gene expression profiling, or genomic testing.

Inside our cells are deoxyribonucleic acid (DNA) molecules. These molecules are tightly packaged into what is called a chromosome. Chromosomes contain most of the genetic information in a cell. Normal human cells contain 23 pairs of chromosomes for a total of 46 chromosomes. Each chromosome contains thousands of genes. Genes are coded instructions for the proteins your cells make. Most genes contain information about a specific protein. A mutation is when something goes wrong in the genetic code. Proteins are given names such as FLT3. Genes are identified in italics like this: *FLT3*.

AML cells sometimes have changes in genes and chromosomes that can be seen under a microscope or found with various other tests.

- Testing of your leukemia cells can gather specific information about your leukemia to help guide treatment.

Leukemia predisposition syndromes

Some hereditary cancer syndromes can be passed down from biological parent to child. A family history of leukemia can affect treatment. A skin punch biopsy might be done if a predisposition condition is suspected. If your blood was tested at diagnosis, you would see the genetic changes of the leukemia. However, these may not be the genetic changes you were born with. Therefore, a skin punch biopsy is used. In this procedure, a small piece of skin and connective tissue is removed to get DNA that hasn't been altered by AML. This will be used to see if you inherited genes that increase your risk of leukemia.

Leukemia predisposition syndrome can affect how your body responds to treatment. Blood and saliva can be used when AML cells disappear (in remission). Biological family members who are possible hematopoietic stem cell donors might be tested for leukemia predisposition syndrome.

While it can be confusing, just know that testing done to look for an inherited gene (germline) mutation or an inherited risk of cancer is different than genetic testing done specifically on cancer cells or testing to look for proteins produced by cancer cells.

- Testing of cells not affected by your leukemia (like skin) can help tell if you have a leukemia predisposition syndrome.

AML mutation testing

A sample of your blood or bone marrow will be studied to see if the AML cancer cells have any specific mutations. This is separate from the genetic testing for mutations that you may have inherited from your biological parents.

AML cells can have changes in genes and chromosomes. Mutation testing using methods such as karyotype, fluorescence in situ hybridization (FISH), polymerase chain reaction (PCR), and next-generation sequencing (NGS) are used to look for these changes or abnormalities. Some mutations may determine the type of treatment given.

There are several different methods by which your blood and bone marrow will be tested for mutations. It is not important for you to know all the different types of mutations or how they happen.

Karyotype

A karyotype is a picture of chromosomes. Normal human cells contain 23 pairs of chromosomes for a total of 46 chromosomes. A karyotype will show extra, missing (deletion), translocated, or abnormal pieces of chromosomes within the leukemia cells. Since a karyotype requires growing cells, a sample of bone marrow or blood must be used.

Karyotype

A karyotype is a picture of your chromosomes.

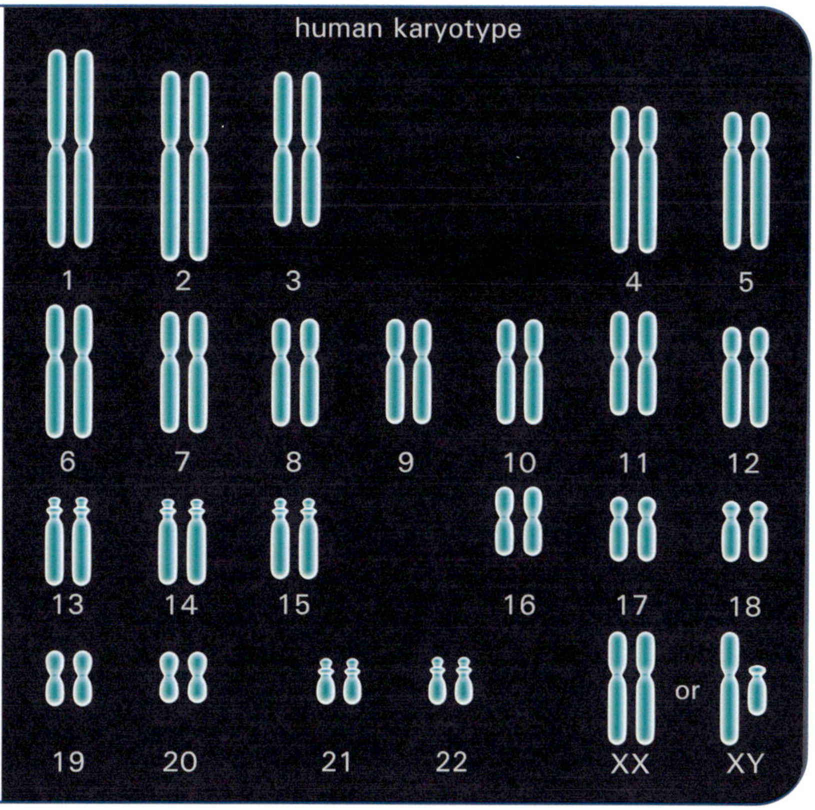

FISH

Fluorescence in situ hybridization (FISH) is a method that involves special dyes called probes that attach to pieces of DNA. FISH can look for changes (abnormalities) that are too small to be seen with other methods. It can only be used for known changes. Since this test doesn't need growing cells, it can be performed on either a bone marrow or blood sample. Sometimes, a bone marrow sample is needed to get all the information the care team needs to help plan your treatment.

PCR

A polymerase chain reaction (PCR) is a lab process that can make millions or billions of copies of one's DNA or RNA (genetic information). PCR is very sensitive. It can find 1 abnormal cell among more than 100,000 normal cells. These copies, called PCR product, might be used for next-generation sequencing (NGS). This is important when testing for treatment response or remission. A real-time or reverse transcriptase (RT) is a type of PCR used to look for gene rearrangements such as *PML::RARA*. This aids in diagnosis and monitoring response to targeted therapies.

Next-generation sequencing

Next-generation sequencing (NGS) is a method used to determine a portion of a person's DNA sequence. It shows if a gene has any mutations that might affect how the gene works. NGS looks at the gene in a more detailed way than other methods and can find mutations that other methods might miss.

AML genetic changes

AML cells can have changes in genes and chromosomes. Mutation testing looks for these changes or abnormalities that are unique to AML cells. Examples of such changes are called deletion, insertion, amplification, translocation (rearrangement), and point mutation.

- ✓ **Amplification** – When a part or whole chromosome or gene is increased (for example, duplicated)
- ✓ **Deletion** – When part of a chromosome or gene is missing such as del(5q)
- ✓ **Insertion** – When a new part of a chromosome or gene is included
- ✓ **Inversion** – Switching of parts within one chromosome such as inv(16) and inv(3)
- ✓ **Point mutation** – When part of a gene is changed
- ✓ **Chromosome translocation and gene rearrangement** – Switching of parts between 2 chromosomes. When described at the chromosome level, it is called a translocation. When described at the gene level, it is called rearrangement. For example, the chromosome translocation is written as t(8;21)(q22;q22.1) and its gene rearrangement is written as *RUNX1::RUNX1T1*.

Imaging tests

In some cases, imaging tests may be performed. It is based on your individual situation. Imaging tests take pictures of the inside of one's body to look for sites with leukemia outside the bone marrow. Leukemia can spread outside the bloodstream to lymph nodes, liver, spleen, and skin. It rarely spreads to the lining of the brain and spinal cord. Imaging tests can also show areas of infection or bleeding that may impact your care.

A radiologist, an expert in interpreting imaging tests, will interpret the test and send the report to your doctor. The doctor will discuss the results with you. While these reports are available to you through your portal, please wait to discuss these results with the doctor.

Contrast material

Contrast material is used to improve the pictures of the inside of the body. Contrast materials are not dyes, but substances that help enhance and improve the images of several organs and structures in the body. It is used to make the pictures clearer. Contrast might be taken by mouth (oral) or given through a vein (IV). The contrast is not permanent and will leave the body in one's urine after the test. The types of contrast vary and are different for CT and MRI. Not all imaging tests require contrast, but many do.

Tell your care team if you have had allergic reactions to contrast in the past. This is important. You might be given medicines to avoid the effects of those allergies. Contrast might not be used if you have a serious allergy or if your kidneys aren't working well.

Brain CT

A computed tomography (CT or CAT) scan uses x-rays and computer technology to take pictures of the same body part from different angles. All the images are combined to make one detailed three-dimensional (3D) picture. A CT of the brain is used to look for bleeding. Contrast should not be used. This is a very quick test.

Brain MRI

A magnetic resonance imaging (MRI) scan uses radio waves and powerful magnets to take pictures of the inside of the body. It does not use x-rays or any radiation. A device will be placed around your head that sends and receives radio waves. An MRI can show if the outer layer of the brain is swollen. Swelling caused by leukemia is called leukemic meningitis. Contrast should be used.

A closed MRI has a capsule-like design where the magnet surrounds you. An open MRI has a magnetic top and bottom, which allows for an opening on each end. Closed MRIs are more common than open MRIs, so if you have claustrophobia (a dread or fear of enclosed spaces), be sure to talk to your care team about it. Also, tell your doctor if there is any metal in your body. MRI scans take longer to perform than CT scans.

PET scan

A positron emission tomography (PET) scan uses a radioactive drug called a tracer. A tracer is a substance injected into a vein to see where cancer cells are in the body and if they are using sugar produced by your body to grow. Cancer cells show up as bright spots on PET scans because they use sugar more quickly than other cells. However, not all cancer cells will appear on a PET scan. Also, not all bright spots are cancer. It is normal for the brain, heart, kidneys, and bladder to be bright on PET. Inflammation or infection can also show up as a bright spot. When a PET scan is combined with CT, it is called a PET/CT scan. An FDG-PET/CT uses a radiotracer called fluorodeoxyglucose (FDG).

Heart tests

Certain treatments can affect heart (cardiac) function. Heart tests are used to see how well your heart works. These tests such as an echocardiogram (echo) or multigated acquisition (MUGA) scan may be needed as a baseline before giving chemotherapy or to monitor treatment side effects. You might be referred to a cardiologist.

Electrocardiogram

An electrocardiogram (ECG or EKG) shows the electrical activity in your heart. It reveals information about your heart rate, rhythm, and electrical conduction. Prolonged corrected QT interval (or QTc) occurs when your heart muscle takes longer than normal to recharge between beats. An ECG is used to detect this. Certain treatments for AML can cause prolonged QTc. If the QTc becomes too prolonged, it can cause dangerous heart rhythms.

Echocardiogram

An echocardiogram (or echo) uses sound waves to make pictures of your heart. For this test, small patches will be placed on your chest to track your heartbeat. Next, a wand (called a transducer) with gel on its tip will be slid across part of your bare chest. A picture of your beating heart will be seen on a screen. The pictures will be recorded for future viewing and interpreted by a cardiologist.

An echocardiogram is one way of measuring ejection fraction, which is the amount of blood pumped out of the left side of your heart every time it beats. This is used to evaluate the function of your heart. In low ejection fraction, the amount of blood pumping from the left side of the heart is lower than normal.

MUGA

A multigated acquisition (MUGA) scan is another way to evaluate the pumping function of your heart. During the test, a small amount of radiotracer will be injected into a vein. A special camera, called a gamma camera, will create computer-generated movie images of your beating heart.

A MUGA scan might show low ejection fraction. This is when the amount of blood pumping from the left side of the heart is lower than normal.

Lumbar puncture

Leukemia can travel to the fluid that surrounds the spine or brain. This may cause symptoms such as headaches, neck pain, and sensitivity to light. To know if leukemia cells are in your spinal fluid, a sample must be taken and tested to rule out a central nervous system (CNS) disease. A lumbar puncture (LP) is a procedure that removes spinal fluid. It is also called a spinal tap. Lumbar punctures are not common in AML.

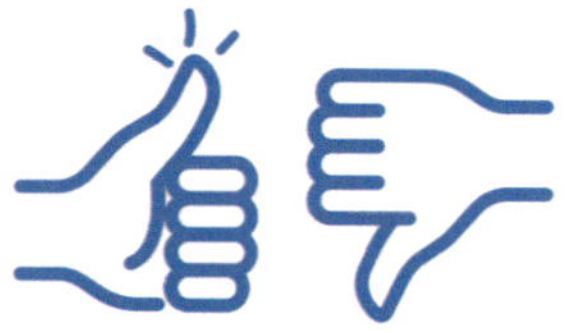

Let us know what you think!

Please take a moment to complete an online survey about the NCCN Guidelines for Patients.

NCCN.org/patients/response

Key points

- Results from blood tests, bone marrow aspirate and biopsy, and imaging studies will determine your treatment plan.
- An aspirate or biopsy is the removal of a sample of tissue or group of cells for testing. A diagnosis of AML is confirmed using a bone marrow aspirate and bone marrow biopsy.
- Genetic and biomarker tests are used to learn more about your type of AML, to target treatment, and to determine the likely path your cancer will take (prognosis).
- HLA typing should be done in those with newly diagnosed AML for whom allogeneic (donor) hematopoietic cell transplant (HCT) is an option.
- Imaging tests are used to look for sites of infection, bleeding, and leukemia that might have spread outside the bloodstream.
- Heart or cardiac tests might be needed to test how well your heart works.
- A lumbar puncture (LP) may be done to look for leukemia in spinal and brain fluid.

Testing takes time. It might take days or weeks for all test results to come in.

3

Treating AML

Treatment for all types of AML will be in phases. The goal of treatment is to put the cancer in remission. This chapter provides an overview of possible treatments and what to expect. Together, you and your care team will choose a treatment plan that is best for your subtype of AML.

Care team

Treating AML takes a team approach. Treatment decisions should involve a multidisciplinary team (MDT). An MDT is a team of health care and psychosocial care professionals from different professional backgrounds who have knowledge (expertise) and experience in your type of cancer. This team is united in the planning and implementing of your treatment. Ask who will coordinate your care.

Some members of your care team will be with you throughout cancer treatment, while others will only be there for parts of it. Get to know your care team and help them get to know you.

Depending on your diagnosis, the care team might include the following specialists:

- **A hematologist or hematologic oncologist** is a medical expert in blood diseases and blood cancers. Other types of oncologists include medical, radiation, and surgical oncologists.
- **A stem cell transplant specialist** oversees the transplantation process, from evaluation to post-transplant care.
- **A pathologist or hematopathologist** analyzes the cells and tissues removed during a biopsy and provides cancer diagnosis. You may never meet this physician in person.
- **Oncology nurses** provide your hands-on care, like giving systemic therapy, managing your care, answering questions, and helping you cope with side effects.
- **Oncology pharmacists** are experts in knowing how to use and dose medicines to treat cancer and to manage symptoms and side effects.
- **Palliative care specialists** concentrate on preventing and alleviating suffering and improving quality of life.
- **Nutritionists and dietitians** can provide guidance on what foods are most suitable for your condition.
- **An occupational therapist** helps people with the tasks of daily living.
- **A physical therapist** helps people move with greater comfort and ease.
- **Psychologists and psychiatrists** are mental health experts who can help manage issues such as depression, anxiety, or other mental health conditions that can affect how you think and feel.

- **Social workers** help people solve and cope with problems in their everyday lives. Clinical social workers also diagnose and treat mental, behavioral, and emotional issues. The anxiety a person feels when diagnosed with cancer might be managed by a social worker in some cancer centers. They, or other designated professionals, can help navigate the complexities of financial and insurance stresses.
- **Spiritual care specialists** identify and support those with spiritual distress or unmet spiritual needs.
- **A research team** helps to collect research data and coordinate care if you are in a clinical trial. Clinical trials help bring new therapies to patients and advance the treatment for everyone. Consider asking your care team about access to clinical trials.

Standard of care is the best-known way to treat a particular disease based on past clinical trials. There may be more than one treatment regimen that is considered standard of care. Ask your care team what treatment options are available and if a clinical trial might be right for you.

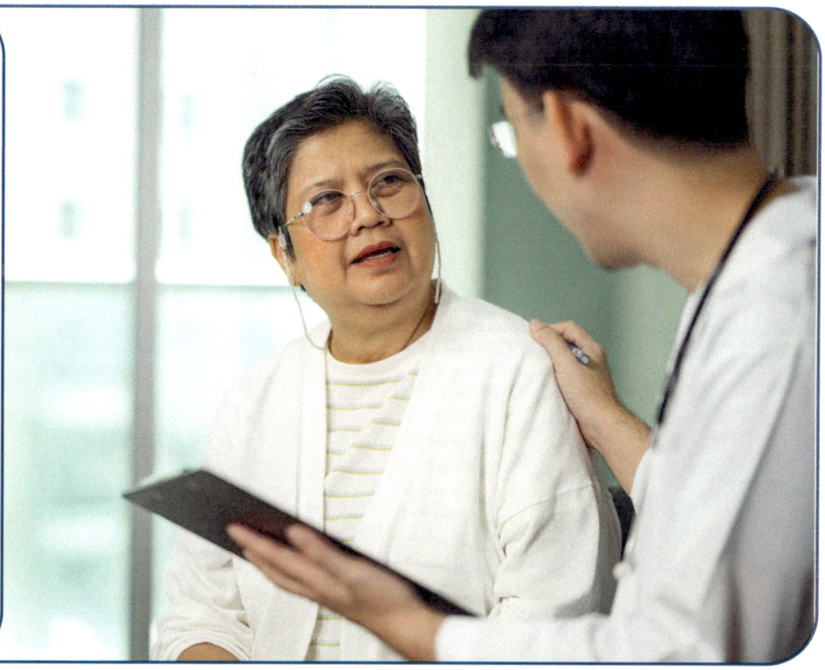

Systemic therapy

Systemic therapy works throughout the body. Types include chemotherapy, targeted therapy, and immunotherapy. Systemic therapy might be used alone or with other therapies. Goals of systemic therapy should be discussed before starting treatment. Your preferences about treatment are important. If you have any religious or personal beliefs about certain kinds of treatment, now would be the time to share them with your care team.

You will likely get either a catheter or a port to deliver systemic therapy, fluids, and blood products into your body. A catheter is a thin, long tube that is often placed in the chest. This goes into a large vein and stays there until treatment is complete. A port is a small, round disc that is usually placed in the chest. The type and location of catheter or port will be tailored to your needs and treatment plans.

Chemotherapy

Chemotherapy is the standard of care for treating AML. Chemotherapy kills fast-dividing cells throughout the body, including cancer cells and normal cells. You will be monitored throughout treatment for side effects or other unwanted (adverse) reactions. All chemotherapy drugs may cause severe, life-threatening, or fatal reactions.

Chemotherapy is most often a liquid that is slowly injected into a vein with a needle. The final dose differs between people because it is based on body weight.

In most cases, chemotherapy is given in cycles of treatment days followed by days of rest. This allows the body to recover before the next cycle. Cycles vary in length depending on which chemotherapy is used. You might spend time in the hospital during treatment.

Types of chemotherapy

There are many types of chemotherapy used to treat AML. Often chemotherapies are combined. This is called multi-agent chemotherapy or a multi-agent regimen. Each chemotherapy works in a different way and causes different side effects. Talk to your care team about the types of chemotherapy you will be given, when you will get them, and what side effects to expect.

Antimetabolites

Antimetabolites prevent the building blocks of DNA from being used. Examples include:

- Cladribine
- Clofarabine (Clolar)
- Cytarabine
- Fludarabine
- Methotrexate

Anthracyclines

Anthracyclines damage and disrupt the making of DNA causing cell death of both cancerous and non-cancerous cells. Some anthracyclines can cause heart issues. They may not be an option for you. There is a limit to how much you can receive in your lifetime. Anthracycline examples include daunorubicin, idarubicin (Idamycin PFS), and mitoxantrone (Novantrone). Dual-drug liposome of cytarabine and daunorubicin (CPX-351 or Vyxeos) includes an antimetabolite and an anthracycline.

Cytarabine

Cytarabine is an anthracycline. Cytarabine (also called Ara-C) is used in many treatment regimens. It might be used alone or in combination with other drugs. It might be given as a single dose to reduce a very high white blood cell count.

There are different doses for cytarabine (Ara-C):

- Standard
- High (HiDAC)
- Intermediate
- Low (LDAC)

The dose you will receive is based on many factors. Ask your care team for the details of your treatment.

- What is the dose?
- How often is treatment received?
- How many treatment cycles are needed?
- Will I need to spend time in the hospital? If so, for how long?

Cytarabine or methotrexate may be used to treat AML in the fluid that surrounds the spine or brain. In this case, it is injected into the spinal fluid. This is called intrathecal chemotherapy.

Hypomethylating agents

Methyl groups are molecules that are found in DNA. They can turn genes on or off. Leukemia cells often have too many methyl groups. These extra groups can block genes from being turned on and off. Hypomethylating agents (HMAs) block methyl groups from binding to DNA. They turn silenced genes back on, which allows leukemic blasts to mature into normal cells. Azacitidine (Vidaza) and decitabine are HMAs.

Targeted therapy

Targeted therapy is a form of systemic therapy that focuses on specific or unique features of cancer cells. Targeted therapies seek out how cancer cells grow, divide, and move in the body. These drugs stop the action of molecules that help cancer cells grow and/or survive.

You will be monitored throughout treatment for side effects or other unwanted (adverse) reactions. As with other systemic therapies, targeted therapy may cause severe, life-threatening, or fatal reactions.

Some examples of targeted therapies:

- Enasidenib (Idhifa)
- Gemtuzumab ozogamicin (GO; Mylotarg)
- Glasdegib (Daurismo)
- Gilteritinib (Xospata)
- Ivosidenib (Tibsovo)
- Midostaurin (Rydapt)
- Olutasidenib (Rezlidhia)
- Quizartinib (Vanflyta)
- Sorafenib (Nexavar)
- Venetoclax (Venclexta)

CD33

Gemtuzumab ozogamicin (GO) is a type of targeted therapy that is linked to a chemotherapy drug. It attaches to a cell surface protein called CD33, then enters the cell. Once inside, chemotherapy is released. Many leukemic blasts have CD33 proteins. Mature blood cells do not have CD33 and are not affected. GO may delay blood count recovery and cause liver issues.

Core binding factor

Core binding factor (CBF) creates a shortage of all types of mature blood cells. Gemtuzumab ozogamicin might be used in combination with daunorubicin and cytarabine to treat AML with CBF or other genetic abnormalities.

FLT3

Gilteritinib or midostaurin is used to treat AML with certain *FLT3* mutations such as *FLT3*-ITD and *FLT3*-TKD. Sorafenib or quizartinib is used to treat AML with an *FLT3*-ITD mutation.

IDH1 and *IDH2*

Ivosidenib and olutasidenib are used to treat AML with an *IDH1* mutation. Enasidenib is used to treat AML with an *IDH2* mutation.

Clinical trials

A clinical trial is a type of medical research study. After being developed and tested in a laboratory, potential new ways of treating cancer need to be studied in people. If found to be safe and effective in a clinical trial, a drug, device, or treatment approach may be approved by the U.S. Food and Drug Administration (FDA).

Everyone with cancer should carefully consider all of the treatment options available for their cancer type, including standard treatments and clinical trials. Talk to your doctor about whether a clinical trial may make sense for you.

Phases

Most cancer clinical trials focus on treatment. Treatment trials are done in phases.

- **Phase 1 trials** study the dose, safety, and side effects of an investigational drug or treatment approach. They also look for early signs that the drug or approach is helpful.
- **Phase 2 trials** study how well the drug or approach works against a specific type of cancer.
- **Phase 3 trials** test the drug or approach against a standard treatment. If the results are good, it may be approved by the FDA.
- **Phase 4 trials** study the long-term safety and benefit of an FDA-approved treatment.

Finding a clinical trial

In the United States

NCCN Cancer Centers
NCCN.org/cancercenters

The National Cancer Institute (NCI)
cancer.gov/about-cancer/treatment/clinical-trials/search

Worldwide

The U.S. National Library of Medicine (NLM)
clinicaltrials.gov

Need help finding a clinical trial?

NCI's Cancer Information Service (CIS)
1.800.4.CANCER (1.800.422.6237)
cancer.gov/contact

Who can enroll?

Every clinical trial has rules for joining, called eligibility criteria. The rules may be about age, cancer type and stage, treatment history, or general health. These requirements ensure that participants are alike in specific ways and that the trial is as safe as possible for the participants.

Informed consent

Clinical trials are managed by a group of experts called a research team. The research team will review the study with you in detail, including its purpose and the risks and benefits of joining. All of this information is also provided in an informed consent form. Read the form carefully and ask questions before signing it. Take time to discuss with family, friends, or others whom you trust. Keep in mind that you can leave and seek treatment outside of the clinical trial at any time.

Start the conversation

Don't wait for your doctor to bring up clinical trials. Start the conversation and learn about all of your treatment options. If you find a study that you may be eligible for, ask your treatment team if you meet the requirements. If you have already started standard treatment you may not be eligible for certain clinical trials. Try not to be discouraged if you cannot join. New clinical trials are always becoming available.

Frequently asked questions

There are many myths and misconceptions surrounding clinical trials. The possible benefits and risks are not well understood by many with cancer.

Will I get a placebo?
Placebos (inactive versions of real medicines) are almost never used alone in cancer clinical trials. It is common to receive either a placebo with a standard treatment, or a new drug with a standard treatment. You will be informed, verbally and in writing, if a placebo is part of a clinical trial before you enroll.

Do I have to pay to be in a clinical trial?
Rarely. It depends on the study, your health insurance, and the state in which you live. Your treatment team and the research team can help determine if you are responsible for any costs.

Hematopoietic cell transplant

A hematopoietic stem cell is an immature cell that can develop into any type of blood cell. A hematopoietic cell transplant (HCT) replaces hematopoietic stem cells that have been destroyed by high doses of chemotherapy and/or radiation therapy as part of the transplant process. You might hear it called a stem cell transplant (SCT) or a bone marrow transplant (BMT). This book will refer to it as HCT. HCTs are performed in specialized centers.

Allogeneic transplant

An allogeneic hematopoietic cell transplant (allogeneic HCT) uses healthy stem cells from a donor. The donor may or may not be related to you. Before an HCT, treatment is needed to destroy bone marrow cells. This is called conditioning and it creates room for the healthy donor stem cells. Your blood will be in a weakened state after conditioning until the donor stem cells settle in and take over as your new blood supply. Conditioning also weakens the immune system so your body won't kill the transplanted cells. Chemotherapy is used for conditioning.

After conditioning, you will receive a transfusion of the healthy stem cells from a donor matched to you. A transfusion is a slow injection of blood products into a vein. This can take several hours. The transplanted stem cells will travel to your bone marrow and grow. New, healthy blood cells will form. This is called engraftment. It usually takes about 2 to 4 weeks. Until then, you will have little or no immune defense. You may need to stay in a very clean room at the hospital or be given antibiotics to prevent or treat infection.

Transfusions are also possible. A red blood cell transfusion is used to prevent bleeding and to treat anemia (below normal red blood cell count). A platelet transfusion is used to treat a low platelet count or bleeding. While waiting for the cells to engraft, you will likely feel tired and weak.

The goal of the transplant is for the new immune system to recognize what remains of the leukemia as foreign and destroy it and to provide you with new, healthy bone marrow.

Possible side effects

Every treatment has side effects. You will be monitored for infections, decreases in your blood counts that require blood transfusions, disease relapse, and graft-versus-host disease (GVHD). In GVHD, the donor cells attack your normal, healthy tissue. There are treatments for GVHD. Ask your care team about the possible side effects or complications of HCT and how this might affect your quality of life.

More information on GVHD can be found at NCCN.org/patientguidelines and on the NCCN Patient Guides for Cancer app.

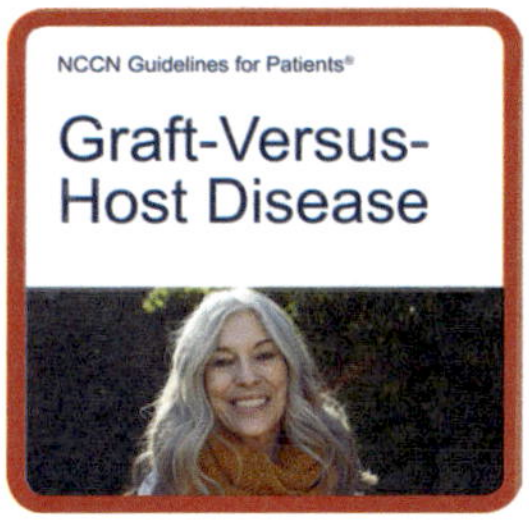

General supportive care

Supportive care will be specific to your needs. Supportive care is health care that relieves symptoms caused by cancer or its treatment and improves quality of life. It might include pain relief, palliative care, emotional or spiritual support, financial aid, or family counseling. Tell your care team how you are feeling and about any side effects so they can be managed. Best supportive care, supportive care, and palliative care often mean the same thing.

It is very important to take care of yourself by eating well, drinking plenty of fluids, exercising, and doing things that make you feel energized.

Side effects

All cancer treatments can cause unwanted health issues called side effects. Side effects depend on many factors. These factors include the drug type and dose, length of treatment, and the person. Some side effects may be harmful to your health. Others may just be unpleasant. AML treatment can cause a number of side effects. Some are very serious.

Ask for a complete list of side effects of your treatments. Also, tell your treatment team about any new or worsening symptoms. There may be ways to help you feel better. There are also ways to prevent some side effects. You will be monitored closely for side effects.

Late effects

Late effects are side effects that occur months or years after a disease is diagnosed or after treatment has ended. Late effects may be caused by cancer or cancer treatment. They may include physical, mental, and social problems, and second cancers. The sooner these effects are treated the better. Ask your care team about what late effects could occur. This will help you know what to look for.

Survivorship

A person is a cancer survivor from the time of diagnosis until the end of life. After treatment, your health will be monitored for side effects of treatment and the return of cancer. This is part of your survivorship care plan. It is important to keep any follow-up doctor visits and imaging test appointments. Seek good routine medical care, including regular doctor visits for preventive care and cancer screening.

A personalized survivorship care plan will contain a summary of possible long-term effects of treatment called late effects and list follow-up tests. Find out how your primary care provider will coordinate with specialists for your follow-up care.

Side effects

Some potential side effects are described next. They are not listed in order of importance. Some side effects are very rare.

Blood clots

Cancer can cause blood clots to form. This can block blood flow and oxygen in the body. Blood clots can break loose and travel to other parts of the body causing breathing problems, stroke, or other problems.

Diarrhea

Diarrhea is frequent and watery bowel movements. Your care team will tell you how to manage diarrhea. It is important to drink lots of fluids.

Distress

Depression, anxiety, and sleeping problems are common and are a normal part of cancer diagnosis. Talk to your care team and with those whom you feel most comfortable about how you are feeling. There are services, people, and medicine that can help you. Support and counseling services are available.

Fatigue

Fatigue is a state of physical or mental tiredness or weakness that can be characterized by a lack of energy, motivation, or stamina. Fatigue may be caused by cancer or it may be a side effect of treatment. Let your care team know how you are feeling and if fatigue is getting in the way of doing the things you enjoy. Eating a balanced diet, exercise, yoga, and massage therapy can help. You

Warnings about supplements and drug interactions

You might be asked to stop taking or avoid certain herbal supplements when on a systemic therapy. Some supplements can affect the ability of a drug to do its job. This is called a drug interaction.

It is critical to speak with your care team about any supplements you may be taking. Some examples include:

- Turmeric
- Ginkgo biloba
- Green tea extract
- St. John's Wort
- Antioxidants

Certain medicines can also affect the ability of a drug to do its job. Antacids, heart or blood pressure medicine, and antidepressants are just some of the medicines that might interact with a systemic therapy or supportive care medicines given during systemic therapy. Therefore, it is very important to tell your care team about any medicines, vitamins, over-the-counter (OTC) drugs, herbals, or supplements you are taking.

Bring a list with you to every visit.

might be referred to a nutritionist or dietitian to help with fatigue.

Infections

Infections occur more frequently and are more severe in those with a weakened immune system. Drug treatment can weaken the body's natural defense against infections.

Neutropenia is very common during leukemia treatment. It is a low number of white blood cells and can lead to frequent or severe infections. When someone with neutropenia also develops a fever, it is called febrile neutropenia (FN). With FN, your risk of infection may be higher than normal. This is because a low number of white blood cells leads to a reduced ability to fight infections. FN is a side effect of some types of systemic therapy. Let your care team know immediately if you are neutropenic and develop a fever.

Loss of appetite

Sometimes side effects from cancer or its treatment, and the stress of having cancer might cause you to feel not hungry or sick to your stomach (nauseated). You might have a sore mouth or difficulty swallowing. Healthy eating is important during treatment. even when you don't have an appetite or get pleasure from eating. It includes eating a balanced diet, eating the right amount of food, and drinking enough fluids. A registered dietitian who is an expert in nutrition and food can help. Speak to your care team if you have trouble eating or maintaining weight.

Low blood cell counts

Some cancer treatments can cause low blood cell counts.

- **Anemia** is a condition where your body does not have enough healthy blood cells, resulting in less oxygen being carried to your cells. You might tire easily if you are anemic.
- **Neutropenia** is a decrease in neutrophils, a type of white blood cell. This puts you at risk for infections that could be dangerous.
- **Thrombocytopenia** is a condition where there are not enough platelets found in the blood. This puts you at risk for bleeding.

Nausea and vomiting

Nausea and vomiting are common side effects of treatment. You will be given medicine to prevent nausea and vomiting.

Neuropathy

Neuropathy is a nerve problem that causes pain, numbness, tingling, swelling, or muscle weakness in different parts of the body. It usually begins in the hands or feet and gets worse over time. Neuropathy may be caused by cancer or cancer treatment. Most of the time, neuropathy goes away after treatment.

Neurotoxicity

Some treatments can damage the nervous system (neurotoxicity) causing problems with concentration, memory, and thinking. Seizures and confusion can occur.

Pain

Tell your care team about any pain or discomfort. You might meet with a palliative care specialist or with a pain specialist to manage pain.

Palliative care

Palliative care is appropriate for anyone, regardless of age, cancer stage, or the need for other therapies. It focuses on physical, emotional, social, and spiritual needs that affect quality of life (QOL).

Quality of life

Cancer and its treatment can affect your overall well-being or quality of life (QOL). For more information on quality of life, see *NCCN Guidelines for Patients: Palliative Care* at NCCN.org/patientguidelines and on the NCCN Patient Guides for Cancer app.

Supportive care resources

More information on supportive care is available at NCCN.org/patientguidelines and on the NCCN Patient Guides for Cancer app.

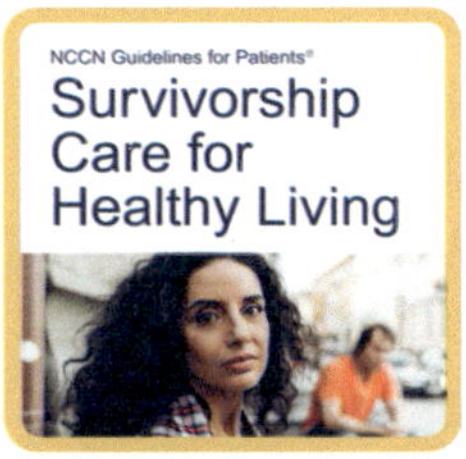

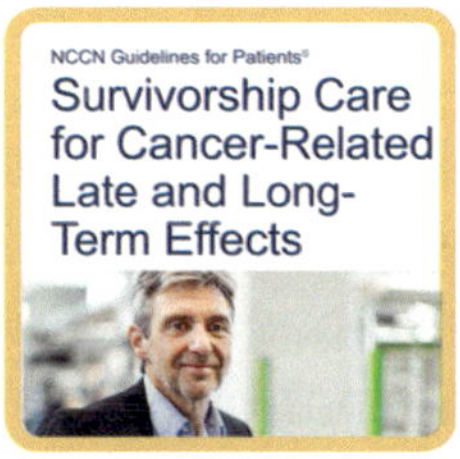

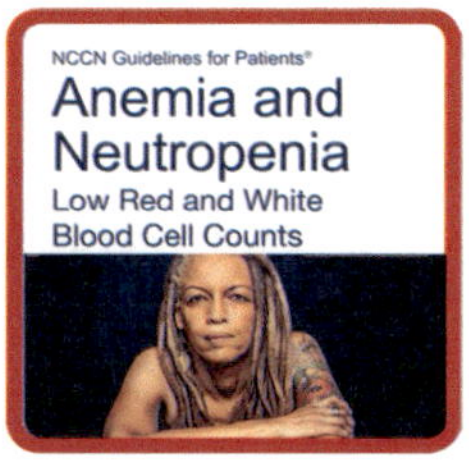

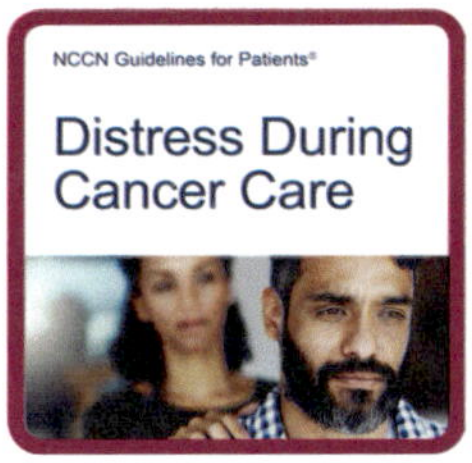

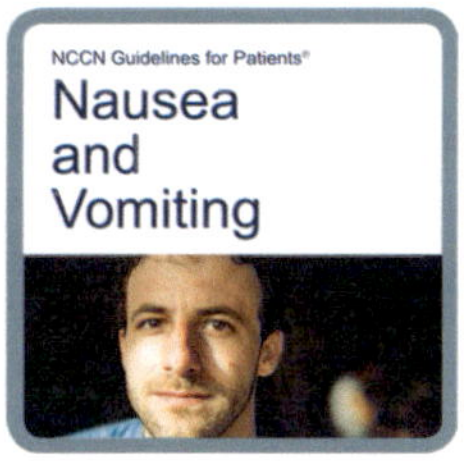

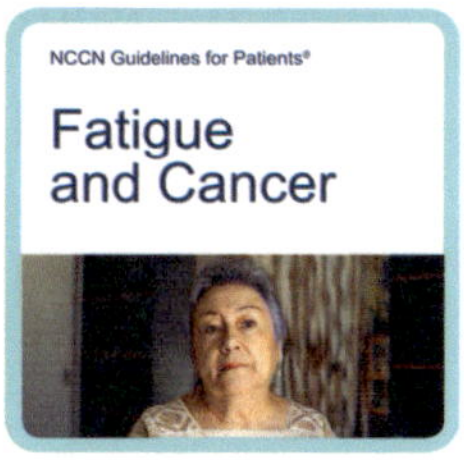

Key points

- A treatment plan is based on your age and other factors such as your overall health and performance status. Performance status is your general level of fitness.
- Systemic therapy works throughout the body. AML is treated with systemic therapy.
- A hematopoietic cell transplant (HCT) aims to restore the body's ability to produce normal blood cells by replacing cancerous bone marrow stem cells with healthy stem cells.
- A clinical trial is a type of research that studies a treatment to see how safe it is and how well it works.
- Supportive care is health care that relieves symptoms caused by cancer or its treatment and improves quality of life. Supportive care is always given.
- All cancer treatments can cause unwanted health issues called side effects. It is important for you to tell your care team about all your side effects so they can be managed.
- It is very important to take care of yourself during treatment by eating well, drinking plenty of fluids, exercising, and doing things that make you feel energized.

All cancer treatments can cause unwanted health issues called side effects. It is important to tell your care team about all of your side effects so they can be managed.

4
AML

There are different types of AML. This chapter is for those with AML that is not APL or BPDCN. It is sometimes referred to as non-APL AML. Together, you and your care team will choose a treatment plan that is best for you.

Overview

There are different types of AML. Most people with leukemia do not have acute promyelocytic leukemia (APL). This chapter is for those with non-APL AML.

Diagnosis

To be diagnosed with AML, myeloblasts must be present in the bone marrow or blood. At diagnosis, most people will have a bone marrow aspirate and biopsy. Some may have a lumbar puncture if there are signs and symptoms of central nervous system (CNS) leukemia.

What causes AML?

AML can happen for certain known reasons, but very often there is no clear cause that can be determined. Certain treatments for other cancers, such as radiation or a certain type of chemotherapy, can later cause AML. Myelodysplastic syndrome (MDS) or other chronic marrow cancers can become AML. MDS is a type of cancer that occurs when bone marrow stops making enough healthy blood cells and abnormal cells are found. AML can also run in certain families, although this is thought to be quite uncommon.

Treatment phases

The goal of the induction phase of treatment is to put AML into complete remission. In complete remission, both bone marrow and blood cell blasts are suppressed, allowing normal marrow function to resume. However, undetected leukemia cells may persist and can return causing relapse. Consolidation therapy, another phase, is needed to prolong remission.

There are different types of treatment responses. When there are no signs of cancer, it is called a complete response (CR) or complete remission (CR). This does not always mean that AML has been cured—there can still be undetectable leukemia cells. Remission can be short-term (temporary) or long-lasting (permanent). Partial remission (PR) and a complete response with partial hematologic (CRh) or incomplete (CRi) blood recovery are also possible. Ask your care team what these terms might mean for your type of AML.

It takes time for bone marrow to make normal blood cells again. This is called recovery. In hypoplasia, bone marrow is starting to recover, but hasn't fully recovered yet.

In complete remission:

- There is no sign of leukemia after treatment.
- Your blood counts have returned to normal.
- You have less than 5 percent (5%) blasts in your bone marrow (or fewer than 5 blasts out of every 100 blood cells).

Treatment for AML can occur over years. The several phases are described next.

Induction

Induction is the first phase of treatment. It is also called remission induction. The goal is to reduce the number of blasts and put AML in remission. As the number of blasts decreases, other types of marrow cells will also decrease. Your marrow will need time to recover, about 4 to 6 weeks, so blood cells can return to normal levels. Treatment attempts to restore the process of making normal blood cells. When blood counts are normal, bone marrow tests will be repeated to see if the leukemia is in remission.

If treatment does not reduce the number of blasts, you may receive more treatment called re-induction. If blasts persist after more induction, treatment options can be found in *Relapsed and refractory disease* on page 46.

Measurable or minimal residual disease

In measurable or minimal residual disease (MRD) very sensitive lab tests, such as PCR, find leukemia cells in your bone marrow. When testing finds MRD, it is called a positive MRD result or MRD positive (MRD+). Ask your care team what this might mean and what the next steps will be.

Consolidation

Your blood will be given time to recover before starting consolidation. Consolidation is the second phase of treatment. It is also called post-remission therapy. Consolidation treats blasts that may have survived induction. Consolidation may be done to prevent relapse while waiting for hematopoietic cell transplant (HCT).

Monitoring

You will have frequent blood tests during induction and consolidation. Bone marrow tests are possible.

Maintenance

For some people, maintenance is the final phase of treatment. The goal is to prolong remission, and the treatment may be received for months to years.

Surveillance

Surveillance watches for any changes in your condition after remission or an hematopoietic cell transplant (HCT). You will have tests during surveillance to check for relapse.

Treatment overview

AML is not treated the same for everyone. As the body ages, it can have difficulty tolerating higher doses or more intense cancer treatments. In addition to age, your overall health, general level of fitness (performance status), and genetic risk play a role in treatment decisions. Some cancers like AML are treated more aggressively than others. An intensive therapy might have more side effects or be of a higher dose than a less intensive therapy. An intensive therapy is not necessarily better. Remission or a complete response (CR) is still possible in lower-intensity treatments.

There are always risks with treatment. Talk with your care team about the risks and why a certain treatment might be better for you. Find out how treatment might affect your quality and length of life. Your preferences about treatment are also important.

Risk groups

ELN2022 refers to the system developed by the European LeukemiaNet (ELN) in 2022 specifically for AML. This system categorizes those with AML into different risk groups based on various factors such as age, cytogenetics (chromosomal abnormalities), molecular genetics (gene mutations), and response to initial treatment. The purpose of this risk classification is to help health care professionals predict the likely course of the disease (prognosis) and tailor treatment strategies accordingly. The ELN2022 risk classification system assists by identifying persons at high-risk who may benefit from more aggressive therapies and persons at low-risk who may require less intensive treatment.

Risk groups are used to make decisions about treatment and to gain information about the likely course your cancer will take. This is called a prognosis. Risk groups will be used in addition to other factors, such as your age and overall health, to plan treatment. **See Guide 2.**

Some treatments are based on risk groups while others are specific to an AML subtype such as:

- Therapy-related AML (AML caused by an earlier treatment for a different cancer)
- Those who had myelodysplastic syndrome (MDS) or chronic myelomonocytic leukemia (CMML) before called antecedent MDS or CMML
- AML with myelodysplasia-related changes called AML-MRC

Guide 2
ELN2022 AML risk groups

Favorable	Includes any of the following abnormal genes: • t(8;21)(q22;q22.1) or *RUNX1::RUNX1T1* • inv(16)(p13.1q22) or t(16;16)(p13.1q22) or *CBFB::MYH11* • Mutated *NPM1* without *FLT3*-ITD • bZIP in-frame mutated *CEBPA*
Intermediate	Includes any of the following abnormal genes: • Mutated *NPM1* with *FLT3*-ITD • Wild-type *NPM1* with *FLT3*-ITD (without adverse-risk genetic lesions) • t(9;11)(p21.3;q23.3) or *MLLT3::KMT2A* • Other abnormalities not classified as favorable or adverse
Poor	Includes any of the following abnormal genes: • t(6;9)(p23;q34.1) or *DEK::NUP214* • t(v;11q23.3) or *KMT2A*-rearranged • t(9;22)(q34.1;q11.2) or *BCR::ABL1* • t(8;16)(p11.2;p13.3) or *KAT6A::CREBBP* • inv(3)(q21.3q26.2) or t(3;3)(q21.3;q26.2) or *GATA2, MECOME(EVI1)* • t(3q26.2;v) or *MECOM(EVI1)-rearranged* • -5 or del(5q) or -7 or -17/abn(17p) • Complex karyotype, monosomal karyotype • Mutated *ASXL1, BCOR, EZH2, RUNX1, SF3B1, SRSF2, STAG2, U2AF1,* and/or *ZRSR2* • Mutated *TP53*

Intensive induction

Favorable and intermediate risk

Intensive induction options for favorable and intermediate risk groups can be found in **Guide 3.**

Guide 3
Favorable and intermediate risk groups: Intensive induction options

Favorable-risk core binding factor (CBF) AML	Preferred: • Standard 7+3 with gemtuzumab ozogamicin (GO) if CD33 positive
	Other recommended: • Standard 7+3 • 7+3 (cytarabine with mitoxantrone) • FLAG-IDA with GO. FLAG-IDA includes fludarabine, high-dose cytarabine (HiDAC), granulocyte colony-stimulating factor (G-CSF), and idarubicin
Favorable-risk *NPM1*, *FLT3* wild-type, or ZIP in-frame *CEBPA* mutations or Intermediate-risk AML	Preferred: • Standard 7+3 • 7+3 (cytarabine with mitoxantrone)
	Other recommended: • Standard 7+3 with GO if CD33 positive • FLAG-IDA • FLAG-IDA with GO if CD33 positive
AML with *FLT3*-ITD mutation	• Standard 7+3 with midostaurin or quizartinib
AML with *FLT3*-TKD mutation	• Standard 7+3 with midostaurin

Poor risk

Intensive induction options for poor risk groups can be found in **Guide 4**.

The standard 7+3 regimen is

- 7 days of cytarabine with
- 3 days of an anthracycline (daunorubicin or idarubicin)

Guide 4
Poor risk groups: Intensive induction options

Therapy-related AML (other than core binding factor AML), antecedent MDS, CMML, or AML-MRC	• CPX-351/dual-drug liposomal cytarabine and daunorubicin • Standard 7+3 • Decitabine with venetoclax • Azacitidine with venetoclax • Low-dose cytarabine (LDAC) with venetoclax • Low-intensity therapy (azacitidine or decitabine) (in some cases)
Poor risk AML	• Clinical trial • Standard 7+3 • CPX-351/dual-drug liposomal cytarabine and daunorubicin • FLAG-IDA (fludarabine, high-dose cytarabine, G-CSF, and idarubicin) • Decitabine with venetoclax • Azacitidine with venetoclax • LDAC with venetoclax • 7+3 (cytarabine with mitoxantrone) • Cytarabine with daunorubicin or idarubicin and etoposide • Low-intensity therapy (azacitidine or decitabine)
Poor risk AML with *TP53* mutation or del(17p) abnormality	• Clinical trial

Less intensive induction

Not everyone wants or can tolerate intensive induction treatment. Age, overall health, and disease features play an important role. Less intensive induction therapy can still cause a complete response (CR). Typically, less intensive chemotherapy will continue indefinitely, as long as it's controlling disease and there is not excess toxicity.

Treatment options are based on the presence or absence of certain actionable gene mutations. An actionable mutation is one that is likely to respond to a targeted therapy.

Guide 5
Less intensive induction options based on mutation

***IDH1* mutation**	Preferred: • Azacitidine with venetoclax • Azacitidine with ivosidenib
	Other recommended: • Decitabine with venetoclax • Ivosidenib
	Used in some cases: • Low-dose cytarabine (LDAC) with venetoclax • Azacitidine or decitabine
Without *IDH1* mutation	Preferred: • Azacitidine with venetoclax • Decitabine with venetoclax
	Other recommended: • LDAC with venetoclax • Azacitidine or decitabine • LDAC with glasdegib • LDAC • Gilteritinib with or without azacitidine (*FLT3*-ITD or TKD mutation) • Azacitidine or decitabine and sorafenib (Sorafenib is used in *FLT3*-ITD mutated AML) • Azacitidine with enasidenib *(IDH2* mutation) • Enasidenib *(IDH2* mutation) • Gemtuzumab ozogamicin (GO) if CD33 positive

Actionable mutations include *IDH1*, *IDH2*, and *FLT3*. Treatment options can be found in **Guide 5.**

After induction

Your next round of induction will be based on which therapy you had first and how AML responded to treatment. Treatment options are based on the amount of cancer or blasts that that remain after induction called measurable or minimal residual disease (MRD). In hypoplasia, bone marrow is starting to recover, but hasn't fully recovered yet. A lumbar puncture might be done. Further treatment is based on if there was a complete response (CR) or less than a complete response to induction.

- **If there was a complete response (remission)**, then treatment might be a cytarabine-based therapy, a continuation of a previous therapy, or a hematopoietic cell transplant (HCT). A clinical trial is also an option, if available and it is what you want.
- **If there was less than a complete response or cancer progressed,** then options include chemotherapy, targeted therapy, a clinical trial, an HCT, or best supportive care. Best supportive care is treatment to improve quality of life and relieve discomfort.

Maintenance

Not everyone will receive maintenance therapy. If given, it will likely be azacitidine, a chemotherapy. For those who had an HCT, then maintenance might be a targeted therapy.

Surveillance

Surveillance is a period of testing that begins after remission to monitor for relapse or the return of cancer. During surveillance, you will have a complete blood count (CBC) every 1 to 3 months for 2 years. After that, a CBC should be repeated every 3 to 6 months for up to 5 years. A bone marrow aspirate and biopsy may be needed.

Relapsed and refractory disease

When leukemia returns it is called a relapse. The goal of treatment is to achieve remission again. You may receive treatment to prevent the blasts from spreading to your brain and spine. A search for a blood stem (hematopoietic) cell donor should begin at first relapse, if this is an option being considered.

When leukemia does not respond to treatment or worsens during treatment, it is called refractory or resistant cancer. The cancer may be resistant at the start of treatment or it may become resistant during treatment. Biomarker testing (including *IDH1*, *IDH2*, and *FLT3* mutations) should be done to determine next treatment options.

For relapsed AML or AML that stops responding to treatment after consolidation, options include:

- Clinical trial (strongly preferred)
- Targeted therapy or chemotherapy followed by an HCT
- Repeat initial successful induction regimen if it's been 12 months or more since the induction regimen
- Best supportive care
- Standard treatment approaches that you have not had before (for example, azacitidine with venetoclax)

Targeted therapy options based on mutation can be found in **Guide 6.**

Guide 6
Targeted therapy based on mutation

AML with *FLT3*-ITD mutation
- Gilteritinib
- Hypomethylating agents (HMAs) such as azacitidine or decitabine with sorafenib

AML with *FLT3*-TKD mutation
- Gilteritinib

AML with *IDH1* mutation
- Ivosidenib
- Olutasidenib

AML with *IDH2* mutation
- Enasidenib

CD33-positive AML
- Gemtuzumab ozogamicin (GO)

Supportive care

Supportive care aims to improve your quality of life. It includes care for health issues caused by cancer or cancer treatment. It is sometimes called palliative care.

All cancer treatments can cause unwanted health issues called side effects. Some side effects are very serious. Ask your treatment team for a complete list of side effects of your treatments. Also, tell your treatment team about any new or worsening symptoms. There may be ways to help you feel better. There are also ways to prevent some side effects.

Supportive care for AML treatment-related side effects is described next.

Abnormal blood cell counts

Before treatment, your white blood cell count may be very high. A high count can cause severe health issues. Apheresis or hydroxyurea can quickly reduce the count. Apheresis is a procedure in which blood is collected, certain types of cells are removed, and your blood is returned to your body.

Blood transfusions

A blood transfusion replaces blood or blood components such as red blood cells or platelets. During treatment, you may need blood transfusions. A blood transfusion is a routine procedure where donated blood is given through a vein in your arm. A blood transfusion typically takes 1 to 4 hours, depending on how much is needed and what part of the blood you need.

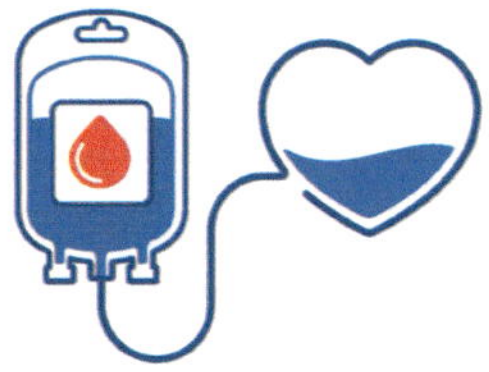

Transfusions

A transfusion is a common procedure to replace blood or blood components (red blood cells or platelets). It is given through an intravenous line (IV), a tiny tube that is inserted into a vein with a small needle.

- ✓ The whole process can take about 1 to 4 hours, depending on how much blood is needed.
- ✓ Most transfusions use blood from a donor.
- ✓ Blood transfusions are usually very safe. Donated blood is carefully tested, handled, and stored.
- ✓ Most people's bodies handle blood transfusions very well. But, like any medical procedure, there are some risks. Speak with your care team for specific information about the risks.
- ✓ Systemic therapy can affect how bone marrow makes new blood cells. Some people getting treatment for cancer might need a transfusion of red blood cells or platelets.

In those with AML receiving a blood transfusion, most of the white blood cells will be removed from donor blood. If treatment will suppress your immune system, then donor blood will also be treated with radiation. These steps will help prevent donor blood from attacking your body. They will also help prevent infections.

Those who do not want blood transfusions

Treatment without blood transfusions is sometimes referred to as bloodless or transfusion-free care. Treatment of AML requires the use of blood and blood products for supportive care. If you do not wish to receive transfusions or certain blood products, please make your wishes known.

If you do not want blood transfusions, your care team will:

- Minimize blood loss and the risk of bleeding
- Discuss goals of care and complications without transfusion
- Ask if certain blood products can be used under certain circumstances
- Discuss if stem cells (from you or a donor who may or may not be related to you) will be acceptable
- Avoid medicines or procedures that can increase the risk of bleeding or myelosuppression. In myelosuppression, bone marrow activity is decreased, resulting in fewer red blood cells, white blood cells, and platelets.

If you do not want blood transfusions, your care team might recommend:

- Vitamin K or other options for those at risk of bleeding or to manage bleeding
- Acetaminophen to manage fever
- Iron, folate, and vitamin B12 supplementation. Iron supplementation may be avoided in someone with excess iron levels.
- Use of erythropoiesis-stimulating agent (ESA), granulocyte colony-stimulating factor (G-CSF), and thrombopoietin (TPO) after a thorough discussion of potential risks, benefits, and uncertainties
- Bed rest and supplemental oxygen in those with severe anemia

Based on your disease, your care team might:

- Test for actionable mutations and consider use of targeted therapies instead of intensive chemotherapy
- Consider use of less myelosuppressive induction including dose reduction of anthracyclines, and use of non-intensive chemotherapy
- Consider referring to centers with experience in bloodless autologous (self) hematopoietic cell transplant (HCT)

Brain issues

Cytarabine can affect the part of the brain that coordinates movement. Symptoms include constant eye movement that can't be controlled. You may be unable to control the range of movement by your legs or arms. Your speech may become slurred.

Differentiation syndrome

Differentiation syndrome is a potentially serious side effect of taking certain anti-cancer drugs. It is caused by a large, fast release of cytokines (an immune protein) as the leukemia cells respond to treatment. Differentiation syndrome used to be called retinoic acid syndrome.

- Symptoms include fever, swelling in limbs, and trouble breathing. You can also gain weight and get a skin rash.
- Signs include low blood pressure and a decrease in blood oxygen levels. Fluid can build up around your lungs or heart. Damage to your kidneys and liver may occur.

Treatment must be started at the first signs or symptoms. Steroids are one effective option for treatment. If there is a rising white blood cell count with differentiation, then an antimetabolite called hydroxyurea (Hydrea) is also frequently used.

Eye issues

High-dose cytarabine may cause the white part of your eyes to become red. Your eyes may feel painful and make more tears. These issues may be prevented with saline or steroid eye drops.

Growth factors

Growth factors, called granulocyte colony-stimulating factor (G-CSF), trigger the bone marrow to make granulocytes (white blood cells). It is sometimes part of an aggressive chemotherapy regimen for relapsed or refractory cancer. Growth factors are an option for supportive care during consolidation if you have a life-threatening infection. Filgrastim (Neupogen) is a G-CSF.

A biosimilar or substitute might be used in place of filgrastim. A biosimilar is almost an identical drug made by another company. It is used in the exact same way and at the same dose as filgrastim.

Infections

If not treated early, infections can be fatal. Infections can be caused by viruses, fungus, or bacteria. Antibiotics can treat bacterial infections. Antifungal medicines can treat fungal infections. You may be given drugs to prevent infections.

Tumor lysis syndrome

In tumor lysis syndrome (TLS), waste released by dead cells builds up in the body causing kidney damage and severe blood electrolyte disturbances. TLS can be life-threatening. Induction chemotherapy may cause TLS. TLS is more likely if your blast count is very high.

Key points

- Chemotherapy is a key part of AML treatment. Targeted therapy may be added if certain gene mutations are present.
- The goal of treatment is a complete response (CR) or remission.
- Measurable or minimal residual disease (MRD) is AML that appears to be in remission, but very sensitive tests find leukemia cells in your bone marrow.
- Leukemia that returns after remission is called relapse.
- When leukemia does not respond to treatment or worsens during treatment, it is called refractory or resistant cancer.
- Supportive care can help to prevent or relieve side effects caused by AML or its treatment and improve quality of life.
- Treatment of AML requires the use of blood and blood products for supportive care. If you do not wish to receive transfusions or certain blood products, please make your wishes known.

Create a medical binder

A medical binder or notebook is a great way to organize all of your records in one place.

- ✓ Make copies of blood tests, imaging results, and reports about your specific type of cancer. It will be helpful when getting a second opinion.
- ✓ Choose a binder that meets your needs. Consider a zipper pocket to include a pen, small calendar, and insurance cards.
- ✓ Create folders for insurance forms, test types (ie, blood, imaging, pathology, radiology, genetics), treatments, and procedures. Organize items in the folder by date.
- ✓ Use online patient portals to view your test results and other records. Download or print the records to add to your binder.
- ✓ Add a section for questions and to take notes.

Bring your medical binder to appointments. You never know when you might need it!

5

APL

In acute promyelocytic leukemia (APL), pieces of chromosomes 15 and 17 break off and trade places creating two fused genes called *PML::RARA* and *RARA::PML*. You will be treated for APL if the *PML::RARA* gene is found. Together, you and your care team will choose a treatment plan that is best for you.

Overview

Acute promyelocytic leukemia (APL) is a rare subtype of AML. About 1 out of every 10 people with AML have APL. Without treatment, APL can worsen quickly and be fatal. With treatment, APL is cured more often than other AML subtypes. APL is treated with all-trans retinoic acid (ATRA) in combination with another systemic therapy.

Diagnosis

The initial diagnosis of APL may be confirmed by a test such as fluorescence in situ hybridization (FISH) or polymerase chain reaction (PCR). APL can be diagnosed quickly, and treatment can be started within just a few hours.

APL usually occurs when parts of chromosome 15 and chromosome 17 break off and trade places, called translocation. This translocation is written as t(15;17). It makes two genes that are fused together. These two fused genes are called *PML::RARA and RARA::PML*. You will be treated for APL if the *PML::RARA* gene is found.

APL can cause bleeding and clotting that can be fatal. You will start taking retinoid (ATRA) right away if your doctor suspects APL. ATRA can stop the bleeding and clotting caused by APL. If tests find you don't have APL, then you will stop taking ATRA.

What causes APL?

In most cases, the causes of APL are not known. Sometimes, certain treatments for other cancers can cause what is known as therapy-related APL.

Treatment phases

Treatment phases for APL include induction and consolidation. Treatment might take place over a period of years. Some types of treatment may be harmful to your heart. Before treatment, your doctor may test how well your heart is working. You may receive treatment for your heart, too.

Treatment response may be measured in the following ways:

- **A hematologic response** measures your blood cell counts.
- **A morphologic response** measures the number of blasts and abnormal cells.
- **A cytogenetic response** measures your chromosomes.
- **A molecular response** measures your molecules (genes).

Induction

Induction is the first phase of treatment. The goal is to reduce the number of blasts and put APL into remission. Treatment is sometimes called remission induction because the focus of induction is remission or a complete response (CR).

In complete remission, there are no signs or symptoms of cancer. It might be more specifically described by the type of remission, such as morphologic or molecular remission. There are different types of complete response or remission. They are described below.

- **A morphologic complete response** occurs when less than 5 percent (5%) blasts are found. This means that less than 5 out of every 100 bone marrow cells are blasts. Induction usually causes a large drop in the number of blasts.
- **A cytogenetic complete response** happens when the translocation of chromosomes 15 and 17 or t(15;17) is no longer found, but the *PML::RARA* gene might still be found.
- **A molecular complete response** will likely follow a cytogenetic response. A molecular response is defined as the absence of the *PML::RARA* gene. This means the *PML::RARA* gene is not found. Often, more treatment (consolidation) is needed to achieve a molecular response.

Treatment needs time to work. Your blood needs time to recover. Blood marrow samples will be taken before starting consolidation. Tests will look for blasts in the marrow. If blasts are absent, induction can be stopped to allow your marrow to make more blood cells.

Consolidation

Consolidation is the second phase of treatment. It treats blasts that may have survived induction. Often, consolidation uses the same drugs as before. Consolidation can cause a long-lasting molecular response. You may have a lumbar puncture before starting consolidation.

Treatment overview

Unlike other types of AML, APL is treated with all-trans retinoic acid (ATRA). Often, ATRA is combined with arsenic trioxide. These treatments are specific to APL. Gemtuzumab ozogamicin (GO), a targeted therapy, might be given. Chemotherapy may also be used.

ATRA

ATRA is made in the body from vitamin A, but it is also made in a lab to treat acne and APL. This drug is also called a retinoid. Retinoid forces APL blasts to mature and become normal cells.

Retinoid is an effective treatment for APL. Used by itself it can achieve a complete response (remission) in most people. However, this response is short-lived. Therefore, other treatments must be added to achieve better results.

Arsenic trioxide (Trisenox)

Arsenic trioxide (or ATO) causes the death of APL cells. When added to ATRA, arsenic trioxide improves treatment outcomes. This means more leukemia cells die and relapse occurs in fewer people. Your heart and electrolytes will be monitored during treatment with arsenic trioxide.

Low-risk group

Those with a white blood cell count of 10 x 109/L (10 billion) or less at diagnosis are placed into the low-risk group. For low risk, the preferred induction therapy option is ATRA with arsenic trioxide. Consolidation will include ATRA with arsenic trioxide.

If arsenic trioxide is not an option, ATRA with idarubicin or gemtuzumab can be used for induction therapy. Consolidation will be a continuation of induction therapy and might include mitoxantrone.

It takes time for blood to recover. You might have a bone marrow biopsy and aspirate before starting consolidation.

High-risk group

Those with a white blood cell count of more than 10 x 109/L (10 billion) at diagnosis are placed into the high-risk group.

Treatment for high risk is based on if you have:

- No heart issues or heart disease
- Heart issues such as low ejection fraction or prolonged QTc

Treatment for high risk is based on those with and without heart issues or heart disease. In all groups, ATRA is used as part of induction therapy. After induction, a bone marrow aspirate and biopsy will be done to look for and confirm remission. A lumbar puncture might be done.

No heart issues

For high risk without heart issues, the preferred induction therapy option is ATRA with arsenic trioxide and either a chemotherapy (idarubicin or cytarabine) or targeted therapy (gemtuzumab). Consolidation will be a continuation of induction therapy and might include mitoxantrone.

High risk with heart issues

For high risk with heart issues such as heart disease, induction options are based on the type of heart issue. All induction options include ATRA. Other systemic therapies might be added. Consolidation will be a continuation of induction therapy. A lumbar puncture is possible.

There are 2 types of heart issues that affect treatment:

- **Low ejection fraction** is when the amount of blood pumping from the left side of the heart is lower than normal. This is measured using a multigated acquisition (MUGA) scan or echocardiogram.
- **Prolonged QT interval (or QTc)** occurs when your heart muscle takes longer than normal to recharge between beats. Often, this electrical disturbance can be seen on an electrocardiogram (ECG).

Monitoring

After completing maintenance therapy, you will enter a monitoring phase. Monitoring is a prolonged period of testing to look for signs that APL has returned, called relapse. PCR tests will be done. Bone marrow or blood samples might be used. You will have no drug therapy during this time.

Relapse

APL can return after remission. A relapse is possible after either a morphologic or molecular response. In relapse after molecular response, the *PML::RARA* gene has returned. You will have bone marrow and genetic tests to confirm you have relapsed APL and not AML caused by previous treatment (called therapy-related AML).

Treatment for first relapse APL will be based on your prior therapy and if it is:

- **Early relapse** (less than 6 months after treatment)
- **Late relapse** (6 or more months after treatment)

The goal of treatment is to achieve remission again. This is not always possible.

Second therapy

After first relapse treatment is complete, your next therapy will be based on if remission was achieved.

- If remission, then the options are a hematopoietic cell transplant (HCT), arsenic trioxide, or a clinical trial.
- You may receive chemotherapy to prevent APL from spreading to your brain and spine (central nervous system or CNS).
- If no remission, then the options are clinical trial or HCT (matched sibling or another donor).

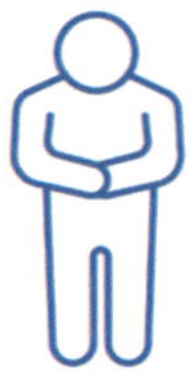

You know your body better than anyone.

Help your care team understand:

- ✓ How you feel
- ✓ What you need
- ✓ What is working and what is not

Keep a list of names and contact information for each member of your team. This will make it easier for you and anyone involved in your care to know whom to contact with questions or concerns.

Get to know your care team and help them get to know you.

Supportive care

Supportive care aims to improve your quality of life. It includes care for health issues caused by cancer or cancer treatment. It is sometimes called palliative care. Palliative care is appropriate for anyone, regardless of age, cancer stage, or the need for other therapies. It focuses on physical, emotional, social, and spiritual needs that affect quality of life (QOL). Tell your treatment team about any new or worsening symptoms.

Supportive care for APL is described next.

Arsenic trioxide monitoring

Arsenic trioxide can cause serious irregular heart rhythms (arrhythmias). You will be monitored for a prolonged QT interval. In prolonged QT, the heart muscle takes longer than normal to recharge between beats. This electrical disturbance often can be seen on an electrocardiogram (ECG).

Bleeding

APL can cause bleeding, or coagulopathy, that can be fatal. Your blood will be tested to see how well it clots. Bleeding can usually be managed with platelet transfusions, cryoprecipitate, and fresh frozen plasma. Cryoprecipitate comes from thawed frozen blood.

Differentiation syndrome

Differentiation syndrome is caused by a large release of cytokines (immune substances) from leukemia cells. Anti-cancer drugs used to treat APL may cause differentiation syndrome. Symptoms of differentiation syndrome include fever, swelling in limbs, and trouble breathing. Weight gain and a skin rash are possible. Signs of differentiation syndrome include low blood pressure and a decrease in blood oxygen. Fluid can build up around your lungs or heart. Damage to your kidneys and liver may occur. This syndrome can be fatal if not caught early.

Seek out support groups at your local hospital, through social media, or from those listed in the back of this book. Look to friends, relatives, neighbors, and coworkers for social support.

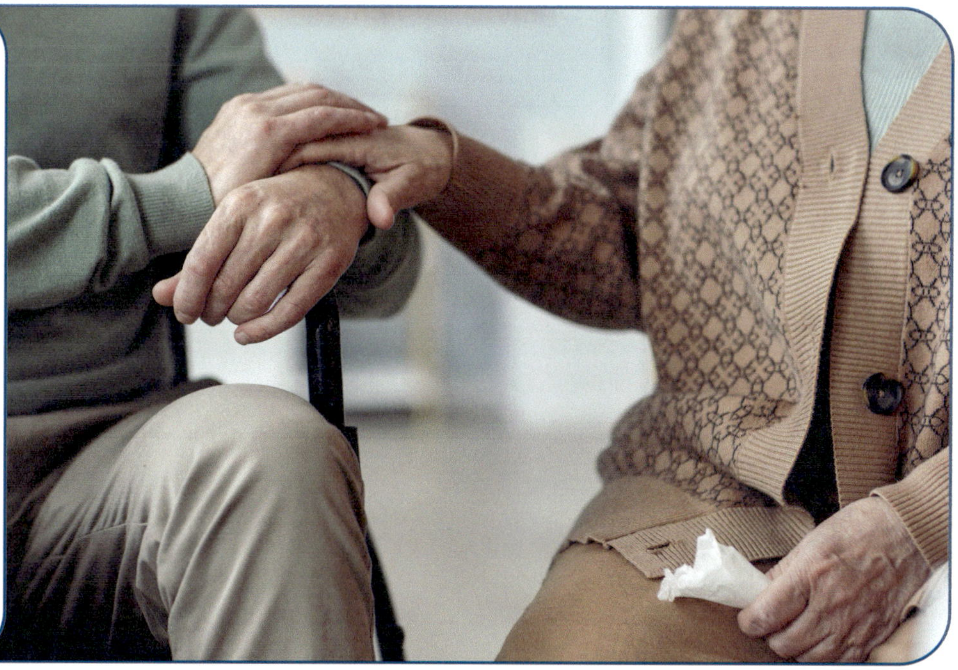

Key points

- Acute promyelocytic leukemia (APL) is a rare subtype of AML. With treatment, APL is cured more often than other AML subtypes.
- APL usually occurs when pieces of chromosomes 15 and 17 break off and trade places creating two fused genes called *PML::RARA* and *RARA::PML*. You will be treated for APL if the *PML::RARA* gene is found.
- APL can cause bleeding that can be fatal. You will start taking retinoid (ATRA) right away if your doctor suspects APL.
- Treatment phases for APL include induction and consolidation. Treatment might take place over a period of years.
- APL is treated with all-trans retinoic acid (ATRA) in combination with another systemic therapy.
- Supportive care aims to improve quality of life and prevent life-threatening health issues caused by APL or its treatment.

Need help paying for medicine or treatment?

Ask your care team what options are available.

6
BPDCN

Blastic plasmacytoid dendritic cell neoplasm (BPDCN) is a very rare, aggressive blood cancer. It is similar to AML. However, unlike AML, BPDCN can be found in blood, bone marrow, lymph nodes, or skin. It is often misdiagnosed. Together, you and your care team will choose a treatment plan that is best for you.

Seek treatment at a cancer center that specializes in BPDCN.

Overview

Blastic plasmacytoid dendritic cell neoplasm (BPDCN) is cancer of the immature plasmacytoid dendritic cells (blasts), a type of immune cell. These blood cells start in the bone marrow and travel to the lymphatic organs such as the spleen and lymph nodes. Skin lesions are common. BPDCN can also affect the central nervous system (CNS).

BPDCN occurs in all races. It is often misdiagnosed because the symptoms and signs vary greatly, and the disease is rare. Therefore, ideally, your treatment team should include doctors from different fields of medicine who are experts in BPDCN.

You might have BPDCN if you have:

- Skin lesions that might be dark purple and large or small spots across the skin. It might look like a rash or bruises. Everyone is different.
- Enlarged lymph nodes
- Stomach pain caused by the disease in the spleen
- Fatigue caused by a decrease in normal blood cells

What causes BPDCN?

Myelodysplastic syndrome (MDS) can become BPDCN. MDS is a type of cancer that occurs when bone marrow stops making enough healthy blood cells and abnormal cells are present. MDS starts in the blood stem cells of bone marrow.

Chronic myelomonocytic leukemia (CMML) can become BPDCN. CMML is a slow-growing type of MDS or myeloproliferative neoplasm (MPN) in which there are too many myelomonocytes, a type of white blood cell, in the bone marrow.

Testing and diagnosis

BPDCN is very difficult to diagnose. It is very important for an expert hematopathologist to review a biopsy when there is concern for BPDCN.

Almost everyone with BPDCN gets skin lesions. BPDCN is often found through a skin biopsy after a visit to the dermatologist for skin lesions. A dermatologist is an expert in the skin. BPDCN may be diagnosed through a lymph node or bone marrow biopsy.

Biomarker and genetic testing will be done to confirm BPDCN and to look for any mutations. Some common gene mutations include *ET2, ASXL1, ZRSR2, SRSF2, TP53, NRAS, IDH2,* and *ETV6.*

For possible tests and procedures, **see Guide 7.**

Treatment overview

BPDCN is a difficult disease to treat. Treatment decisions should involve a multidisciplinary team of doctors from different fields of medicine, including a dermatologist, who are experienced in treating BPDCN.

Treatment for BPDCN includes tagraxofusp-erzs (preferred) or high-dose chemotherapy followed by hematopoietic cell transplant (HCT). Not everyone can tolerate this approach. BPDCN usually returns (relapses) soon after treatment.

Guide 7 Possible tests and procedures: BPDCN
Medical history and physical exam
Complete blood count (CBC), platelets, differential, and comprehensive metabolic panel (CMP)
Analysis of skin lesions (your doctor should work with a dermatologist), blood, bone marrow, and lymph nodes
Bone marrow aspirate and biopsy with lymph node biopsy
BPDCN biomarker and genetic testing
FDG-PET/CT, if leukemia suspected outside the blood and bone marrow (extramedullary) or in lymph nodes
Lumbar puncture (LP)

Intensive therapy

The goal of intensive therapy is to put BPDCN into remission (to achieve a complete response [CR]). Intensive therapy is not for everyone. Treatment will be based on factors such as your overall health and your body's ability to tolerate drug therapies that could be toxic. Your wishes are also important. Talk with your care team about what to expect from treatment and what you want from treatment.

Tagraxofusp-erzs (preferred)

Tagraxofusp-erzs (Elzonris) is a biologic therapy. A biologic is made from a living organism or its by-product like in a vaccine. It helps to improve the body's natural response against cancer.

Tagraxofusp-erzs targets the CD123 protein marker found at higher levels on BDPCN cancer cells. This leads to cancer cell death. You must be in good overall health to receive this treatment. Tagraxofusp-erzs can cause harmful side effects.

The first cycle of this drug should be given in a hospital where it is recommended you stay for at least 24 hours after the treatment is complete. This is to monitor for toxicity and to treat side effects. You will probably spend more than one week in the hospital.

Chemotherapy

There are 3 chemotherapy induction options:

- Cytarabine with idarubicin or daunorubicin
- HyperCVAD
- CHOP (cyclophosphamide, doxorubicin, vincristine, and prednisone)

In hyperCVAD chemotherapy, treatment alternates between two groups of drugs. Hyper means chemotherapy is given in smaller doses and more often to minimize side effects.

Your preferences about treatment are always important. If you have any religious or personal beliefs about certain kinds of treatment, share them with your care team and make your wishes known.

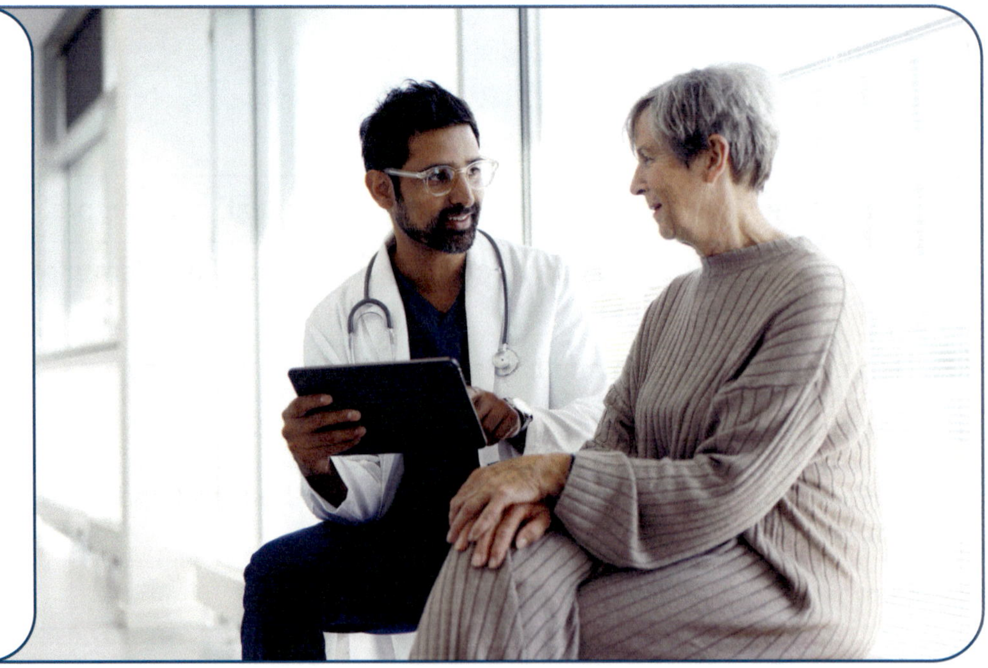

CVAD stands for the first group of drugs: cyclophosphamide, vincristine, doxorubicin (also known by its trade name, Adriamycin), and dexamethasone. The second group of drugs consists of methotrexate and cytarabine. Sometimes, other drugs are added.

Complete remission

After a complete response (CR), options are to continue tagraxofusp-erzs until disease progression or consider a hematopoietic cell transplant (HCT). After an HCT, you will enter surveillance. Surveillance is a plan that closely watches your condition. You might hear it called watch-and-wait. During this time, you will have tests on a regular basis to look for changes in your blood. You will not have any treatment during surveillance.

Surveillance includes a complete blood count (CBC) every 1 to 3 months for 2 years, then every 3 to 6 months for up to 5 years. You might have a bone marrow aspirate and biopsy. You might also have an FDG-PET/CT if you had extramedullary disease before. This is cancer that might be in the lymph nodes or other organs. Skin or other lesions might be biopsied.

Less than complete remission

If BPDCN does not seem to be responding to treatment or there is less than a complete response, then it will be treated as refractory disease. If the skin still shows microscopic disease (CRc), you might have more cycles (at least 4) of therapy before starting treatment for refractory disease.

No intensive therapy

If intensive therapy is not an option, then treatment options are based on whether BPDCN is systemic or localized. In both cases, treatment is to palliate or to give relief.

Localized disease

If BPDCN is found only in the skin or isolated to a certain area of the body, then treatment will focus on those areas. It might include radiation therapy to the lesion(s) or surgery to remove lesions.

Systemic disease

Systemic means the cancer is throughout the body. Treatment includes venetoclax-based therapy, systemic steroids, and supportive care. Venetoclax-based therapy is a low-intensity targeted therapy.

Relapsed and refractory disease

When leukemia returns, it is called a relapse. The goal of treatment is to achieve remission again. You may receive treatment to prevent the blasts from spreading to your brain and spine. Relapse is common in BPDCN. Not everyone's cancer responds to treatment in the same way.

When leukemia does not respond to treatment or progresses during treatment, it is called refractory or resistant cancer. The cancer may be resistant at the start of treatment or it may become resistant during treatment.

A clinical trial is the preferred treatment for relapsed and refractory BPDCN. Tagraxofusp-erzs (Elzonris) is also a preferred option if it was not used before. Other options include systemic therapy or radiation. **See Guide 8.**

Supportive care

Supportive care is health care that relieves your symptoms caused by cancer and improves your quality of life. It is not cancer treatment. In BPDCN, supportive care might include radiation therapy or surgery to treat skin lesions. Everyone with BPDCN should have a dermatologist as part of their care team.

Dermatologist

It is important to see an experienced dermatologist and that your doctors work together on your treatment.

Guide 8 Treatment options: Relapsed and refractory BPDCN
Evaluate central nervous system (CNS) for disease
Clinical trial (preferred)
Tagraxofusp-erzs (preferred if not used before) with supportive care
Chemotherapy (if not already used)
Local radiation to isolated areas or specific lesions
Systemic steroids
Venetoclax-based therapy
Start a donor search at first relapse for those who are candidates for a hematopoietic cell transplant (HCT) with no sibling donor match

Tagraxofusp-erzs

Tagraxofusp-erzs can have very serious side effects. You will have blood tests to closely monitor your health. Capillary leak syndrome and hypoalbuminemia are serious and life-threatening conditions that can occur if you take tagraxofusp-erzs.

Capillary leak syndrome

Tagraxofusp-erzs injection may cause a serious and life-threatening reaction called capillary leak syndrome. In capillary leak syndrome, fluid and proteins leak out of tiny blood vessels causing dangerously low blood pressure. This may lead to organ failure and death. You will be monitored for capillary leak syndrome. You might be asked to weigh yourself every day while taking tagraxofusp-erzs. Sudden weight gain might be a sign of capillary leak syndrome.

Hypoalbuminemia

Hypoalbuminemia is a medical sign that protein levels of albumin are too low in the blood. It is most often the result of capillary leak syndrome.

Key points

- Blastic plasmacytoid dendritic cell neoplasm (BPDCN) is a rare, aggressive blood cancer of immature plasmacytoid dendritic cells, a type of immune cell.
- BPDCN affects the blood, bone marrow, and skin. It can also affect the lymph nodes, spleen, and central nervous system (CNS).
- BPDCN is often found through a skin biopsy after a visit to the dermatologist for skin lesions.
- BPDCN is treated with a biologic therapy called tagraxofusp-erzs or with a combination of chemotherapies. A hematopoietic cell transplant (HCT) might follow treatment.
- Capillary leak syndrome and hypoalbuminemia are serious and life-threatening conditions that can occur if you take tagraxofusp-erzs.
- A clinical trial is the preferred treatment for relapsed and refractory BPDCN.

7

Making treatment decisions

It's important to be comfortable with the cancer treatment you choose. This choice starts with having an open and honest conversation with your care team.

It's your choice

In shared decision-making, you and your care team share information, discuss the options, and agree on a treatment plan. It starts with an open and honest conversation between you and your care team.

Treatment decisions are very personal. What is important to you may not be important to someone else. Some things that may play a role in your decision-making:

- What you want and how that might differ from what others want
- Your religious and spiritual beliefs
- Your feelings about certain treatments
- Your feelings about pain or side effects
- Cost of treatment, travel to treatment centers, and time away from school or work
- Quality of life and length of life
- How active you are and the activities that are important to you

Think about what you want from treatment. Discuss openly the risks and benefits of specific treatments and procedures. Weigh options and share concerns with your care team. If you take the time to build a relationship with your care team, it will help you feel supported when considering options and making treatment decisions.

Second opinion

It is normal to want to start treatment as soon as possible. While cancer can't be ignored, there is time to have another doctor review your test results and suggest a treatment plan. This is called getting a second opinion, and it's a normal part of cancer care. Even doctors get second opinions!

Things you can do to prepare:

- Check with your insurance company about its rules on second opinions. There may be out-of-pocket costs to see doctors who are not part of your insurance plan.
- Make plans to have copies of all your records sent to the doctor you will see for your second opinion.

Support groups

Many people diagnosed with cancer find support groups to be helpful. Support groups often include people at different stages of treatment. Some people may be newly diagnosed, while others may be finished with treatment. If your hospital or community doesn't have support groups for people with cancer, check out the websites listed in this book.

Questions to ask

Possible questions to ask your care team are listed on the following pages. Feel free to use these questions or come up with your own.

Questions about diagnosis and testing

1. What subtype of AML do I have? What does this mean in terms of my prognosis and treatment options?

2. What tests do I need? What other tests do you recommend?

3. How soon will I know the results and who will explain them to me?

4. Where will the tests take place? How long will the tests take?

5. Will treatment start before the test results are in?

6. Is there a cancer center or hospital nearby that specializes in my type and subtype of cancer?

7. What will you do to make me comfortable during testing?

8. Would you give me a copy of the pathology report and other test results?

9. Who will talk with me about the next steps? When?

10. How many bone marrow tests are needed? When are they done?

Questions about options

1. What will happen if I do nothing?
2. Am I a candidate for a hematopoietic cell transplant (HCT)?
3. Am I a candidate for a clinical trial?
4. Can I join a clinical trial at any time?
5. Which option is proven to work best for my cancer, age, health, and other factors?
6. Can I stop treatment at any time? What will happen if I stop treatment?
7. What are my options if treatment doesn't work as expected?
8. How will I know when blood transfusions or antibiotics are needed?
9. What decisions must be made today? Is there a social worker or someone who can help me decide?
10. Is there a hospital or treatment center you can recommend for treatment?

Questions about treatment

1. Which treatment do you recommend and why?
2. Which treatment will give me the best quality of life?
3. Which treatment will extend life? By how long?
4. What should I expect from this treatment?
5. When will I start treatment?
6. How long will treatment take?
7. How much will my insurance pay for this treatment?
8. What are the chances my cancer will return?
9. How will my cancer be treated if it returns?
10. How long will treatment last?

Questions about your care team's experience

1. What is your experience treating AML?
2. What is the experience of those on your team?
3. What other types of cancer do you treat?
4. I would like another pathologist or hemopathologist to review my blood samples. Is there someone you recommend?
5. How many people like me (of the same age, gender, race) have you treated?
6. Will you be consulting with AML experts to discuss my health care? Whom will you consult?
7. How many procedures like the one you're suggesting have you done?
8. Is this treatment a major part of your practice?
9. How many of your patients have had complications? What were the complications?
10. Who will manage my day-to-day care?

Questions about side effects

1. What are the side effects of this treatment?
2. How long will these side effects last?
3. Do any side effects lessen or worsen in severity over time?
4. What side effects are expected and which are life threatening?
5. When should I call the doctor? Can I text?
6. What should I do for an issue on weekends and other non-office hours?
7. What medicines can I take to prevent or relieve side effects?
8. Will you stop treatment or change treatment if there are side effects? What do you look for?
9. What can I do to lessen or prevent side effects? What will you do?
10. What side effects are life-long and irreversible even after completing treatment?

Questions about blood transfusions

1. How often will I need blood transfusions?
2. How long does a transfusion take?
3. How will I feel after a transfusion?
4. Can I be given blood donated by family members?
5. Should my friends and family donate blood?
6. What are the side effects of blood transfusions?
7. Can my body reject blood transfusions? Is this serious?
8. If my body rejects a blood transfusion, will I be able to have more blood transfusions?

Questions about radiation therapy

1. What type of radiation therapy (RT) will I have?
2. What will you target?
3. What is the goal of this RT?
4. How many treatment sessions will I need?
5. Can you do a shorter course of RT?
6. Do you offer this type of RT here? If not, should you refer me to someone who does?
7. What side effects can I expect from RT?
8. Will I be given medicine to help me relax during RT?
9. What should I wear?

Questions about hematopoietic cell transplants

1. Which type of hematopoietic cell transplant (HCT) is an option for me?
2. How do you find a donor?
3. What are the risks to myself and/or the donor?
4. How will an HCT affect my prognosis?
5. How will an HCT affect the quality and length of my life?
6. How long should I expect to be in the hospital?
7. How will I feel before, during, and after the HCT?
8. How many HCTs has this center done for my type of AML?
9. Will I have more than one HCT?
10. What side effects may occur after an HCT?

Questions about clinical trials

1. What clinical trials are available?
2. What are the treatments used in the clinical trial?
3. What does the treatment do?
4. Has the treatment been used before? Has it been used for other types of cancer?
5. What are the risks and benefits of this treatment?
6. What side effects should I expect?
7. How will the side effects be controlled?
8. How long will I be in the clinical trial?
9. Will I be able to get other treatment if this doesn't work?
10. Will the clinical trial cost me anything? If so, how much?

Questions about resources and support

1. Who can I talk to about help with housing, food, and other basic needs?
2. What help is available for transportation, childcare, and home care?
3. How much will I have to pay for treatment?
4. What help is available to pay for medicines and other treatment?
5. What other services are available to me and my caregivers?
6. How can I connect with others and build a support system?
7. How can I find in-person or online support?
8. Who can help me with my concerns about missing work or school?
9. Who can I talk to if I don't feel safe at home, at work, or in my neighborhood?
10. How can I get help to stop smoking or vaping?

Resources

Be the Match
bethematch.org/one-on-one

Blood & Marrow Transplant Information Network (BMT InfoNet)
bmtinfonet.org

Cancer*Care*
cancercare.org

Cancer Hope Network
cancerhopenetwork.org

MedlinePlus
medlineplus.gov

National Cancer Institute (NCI)
cancer.gov/types/leukesmia

National Bone Marrow Transplant Link (nbmtLINK)
nbmtlink.org

National Coalition for Cancer Survivorship
canceradvocacy.org

The Leukemia & Lymphoma Society
LLS.org/PatientSupport

Triage Cancer
triagecancer.org

Words to know

acute myeloid leukemia (AML)
A fast-growing cancer of young white blood cells called myeloblasts.

acute promyelocytic leukemia (APL)
A fast-growing subtype of AML.

allogeneic
Donor who may or may not be related to you.

all-trans retinoic acid (ATRA)
ATRA is made in the body from vitamin A. ATRA made in a lab is used to treat APL.

anemia
A health condition in which the number of red blood cells is low.

antimetabolite
A drug that interferes with normal cell division and cell function.

arsenic trioxide (ATO)
A drug used to treat APL that has a fusion gene *PML::RARA*.

autologous
Stem cells come from you.

best supportive care
Treatment to improve quality of life and relieve discomfort.

biomarker testing
A lab test of any molecule in your body that can be measured to assess your health. Also called molecular testing.

blast
An immature white blood cell. Also called a myeloblast.

blastic plasmacytoid dendritic cell neoplasm (BPDCN)
A rare, aggressive blood cancer that has features of leukemia, lymphoma, and skin cancer.

blood stem cell
A blood-forming cell from which all other types of blood cells are formed. Also called hematopoietic stem cell.

bone marrow
The sponge-like tissue in the center of most bones where blood cells are made.

bone marrow aspirate
The removal of a small amount of liquid bone marrow to test for a disease.

bone marrow biopsy
The removal of a small amount of solid bone and bone marrow to test for a disease.

chemotherapy
Drugs that kill fast-dividing cells, including cancer cells and normal cells.

chromosome
Long strands that contain bundles of coded instructions for making and controlling cells.

complete response (CR)
An absence of all signs and symptoms of cancer after treatment. Also called complete remission.

computed tomography (CT)
A test that uses x-rays from many angles to make a picture of the insides of the body.

consolidation
A shorter and more intense treatment phase to further reduce the number of cancer cells. It is the second phase of treatment.

contrast
A substance put into your body to make clearer pictures during imaging tests.

core binding factor (CBF) AML
A form of AML that creates a shortage of all types of mature blood cells.

cytogenetic complete response
The absence of t(15;17) after treatment for acute promyelocytic leukemia (APL).

cytogenetics
The study of chromosomes using a microscope.

cytopenia
A health condition when the number of blood cells is lower than normal.

deoxyribonucleic acid (DNA)
Long strands of genetic information found inside cells.

differential
A lab test of the number of white blood cells for each type.

differentiation syndrome
A group of health signs and symptoms that is caused by leukemia or its treatments.

extramedullary
Outside the bone marrow.

flow cytometry (FCM)
A lab test of substances on the surface of cells to identify the type of cells present.

fluorescence in situ hybridization (FISH)
A lab test that uses special dyes to look for abnormal chromosomes and genes.

fusion gene
A gene that is made when parts of two separate genes join.

gene
A set of coded instructions in cells for making new cells and controlling how cells behave.

graft-versus-host disease (GVHD)
A disease that occurs when transplanted blood stem cells attack a patient's normal cells.

hematologist
A doctor who's an expert in diseases of the blood.

hematopathologist
A doctor who specializes in the study of blood diseases and cancers using a microscope.

hematopoietic cell
An immature blood-forming cell from which all blood cells are formed. Also called blood stem cell.

hematopoietic cell transplant (HCT)
A treatment that replaces damaged or diseased cells in the bone marrow with healthy blood-forming cells. Also called stem cell transplant (SCT) or bone marrow transplant (BMT).

hereditary
Passed down from biological parent to child through coded information in cells (genes).

human leukocyte antigen (HLA)
Special proteins on the surface of cells that help the body to tell its own cells apart from foreign cells.

immunohistochemistry (IHC)
A lab test used to find specific cell traits.

immunophenotyping
A lab test that detects the type of cells present based on the cells' surface proteins.

induction
The first phase of treatment.

lumbar puncture (LP)
A procedure that removes spinal fluid with a needle. Also called a spinal tap.

magnetic resonance imaging (MRI)
A test that uses radio waves and powerful magnets to make pictures of the insides of the body.

maintenance
Usually the last treatment phase given to prolong treatment results.

medullary
In the bone marrow.

molecular complete response
The absence of the *PML::RARA* gene after treatment for acute promyelocytic leukemia (APL).

morphologic complete response
A large decrease in number or percent of blasts after treatment for acute leukemia.

mutation
An abnormal change.

myeloid
Referring to a type of white blood cell called a granulocyte.

myelosuppression
A condition in which bone marrow activity is decreased, resulting in fewer red blood cells, white blood cells, and platelets.

pathologist
A doctor who's an expert in testing cells and tissue to find disease.

peripheral blood
Blood that circulates throughout the body.

platelet (PLT)
A type of blood cell that helps control bleeding. Also called thrombocyte.

polymerase chain reaction (PCR)
A lab process in which copies of a piece of DNA are made.

positron emission tomography (PET)
A test that uses radioactive material to see the shape and function of body parts.

prognosis
The likely course and outcome of a disease.

progression
The growth or spread of cancer during or after treatment.

recovery
A period of time without treatment to allow blood cell counts to return to normal.

red blood cell (RBC)
A type of blood cell that carries oxygen from the lungs to the rest of the body. Also called an erythrocyte.

refractory
A cancer that does not improve with treatment.

regimen
A treatment plan that includes specific information about drug dose, when medicine is taken, and how long treatment will last.

relapse
The return or worsening of cancer after a period of improvement.

remission
There are minor or no signs of a disease.

resistance
When cancer does not respond to a drug treatment.

side effect
An unhealthy or unpleasant physical or emotional response to treatment.

standard of care
The best-known way to treat a particular disease based on past clinical trials. There may be more than one treatment regimen that is considered standard of care.

subtype
A smaller group within a type of cancer that is based on certain cell features.

supportive care
Health care that includes symptom relief but not cancer treatment. Also called palliative care or best supportive care.

surveillance
Testing that is done after treatment ends to check for the return of cancer.

systemic therapy
Treatment that works throughout the body.

targeted therapy
A drug treatment that targets and attacks specific cancer cells.

translocation
When pieces of two chromosomes (long strands of coded instructions for controlling cells) break off and switch with each other.

tumor lysis syndrome (TLS)
A condition caused when waste released by dead cells is not quickly cleared out of your body.

white blood cell (WBC)
A type of blood cell that helps fight infections in the body. Also called a leukocyte.

share with us.

Take our survey and help make the NCCN Guidelines for Patients better for everyone!

NCCN.org/patients/comments

NCCN Contributors

This patient guide is based on the NCCN Clinical Practice Guidelines in Oncology (NCCN Guidelines®) for Acute Myeloid Leukemia, Version 1.2024. It was adapted, reviewed, and published with help from the following people:

Dorothy A. Shead, MS
Senior Director
Patient Information Operations

Tanya Fischer, MEd, MSLIS
Senior Medical Writer

Laura Phillips
Graphic Artist

The NCCN Clinical Practice Guidelines in Oncology (NCCN Guidelines®) for Acute Myeloid Leukemia, Version 1.2024 were developed by the following NCCN Panel Members:

*Daniel A. Pollyea, MD, MS/Chair
University of Colorado Cancer Center

Jessica K. Altman, MD/Vice Chair
Robert H. Lurie Comprehensive Cancer Center of Northwestern University

*Rita Assi, MD
Indiana University Melvin and Bren Simon Comprehensive Cancer Center

*Kimo Bachiashvili, MD, MPH
O'Neil Comprehensive Cancer Center at UAB

Amir T. Fathi, MD
Mass General Cancer Center

James M. Foran, MD
Mayo Clinic Comprehensive Cancer Center

Ivana Gojo, MD
The Sidney Kimmel Comprehensive Cancer Center at Johns Hopkins

Aaron Goldberg, MD, PhD
Memorial Sloan Kettering Cancer Center

Aric C. Hall, MD
University of Wisconsin Carbone Cancer Center

Brian A. Jonas, MD, PhD
UC Davis Comprehensive Cancer Center

Ashwin Kishtagari, MD
Vanderbilt-Ingram Cancer Center

Jeffrey Lancet, MD
Moffitt Cancer Center

*Matthew Levine, MD
Patient Advocate

Lori Maness, MD
Fred & Pamela Buffett Cancer Center

James Mangan, MD, PhD
UC San Diego Moores Cancer Center

Gabriel Mannis, MD
Stanford Cancer Institute

Guido Marcucci, MD
City of Hope National Medical Center

Alice Mims, MD, MS
The Ohio State University Comprehensive Cancer Center - James Cancer Hospital and Solove Research Institute

Kelsey Moriarty, MS, CGC
UT Southwestern Simmons Comprehensive Cancer Center

Moaath Mustafa Ali, MD, MPH
Case Comprehensive Cancer Center/ University Hospitals Seidman Cancer Center and Cleveland Clinic Taussig Cancer Institute

Jadee Neff, MD, PhD
Duke Cancer Institute

Reza Nejati, MD
Fox Chase Cancer Center

Rebecca Olin, MD, MSCE
UCSF Helen Diller Family Comprehensive Cancer Center

*Anand Patel, MD
The UChicago Medicine Comprehensive Cancer Center

Mary-Elizabeth Percival, MD, MS
Fred Hutchinson Cancer Center

Alexander Perl, MD
Abramson Cancer Center at the University of Pennsylvania

Kristen Pettit, MD
University of Michigan Rogel Cancer Center

Amanda Przespolewski, DO
Roswell Park Comprehensive Cancer Center

Dinesh Rao, MD, PhD
UCLA Jonsson Comprehensive Cancer Center

Farhad Ravandi, MD
The University of Texas MD Anderson Cancer Center

*Rory Shallis, MD
Yale Cancer Center/Smilow Cancer Hospital

Paul J. Shami, MD
Huntsman Cancer Institute at the University of Utah

Richard M. Stone, MD
Dana-Farber/Brigham and Women's Cancer Center

Swapna Thota, MD
St. Jude Children's Research Hospital/ The University of Tennessee Health Science Center

Geoffrey Uy, MD
Siteman Cancer Center at Barnes-Jewish Hospital and Washington University School of Medicine

NCCN

Ajibola Awotiwon, MBBS, MSc
Guidelines Layout Specialist

Carly J. Cassara, MSc
Guidelines Layout Specialist

Katie Stehman, PA-C, MMS
Oncology Scientist/Medical Writer

* Reviewed this patient guide. For disclosures, visit NCCN.org/disclosures.

NCCN Cancer Centers

Abramson Cancer Center
at the University of Pennsylvania
Philadelphia, Pennsylvania
800.789.7366 • *pennmedicine.org/cancer*

Case Comprehensive Cancer Center/
University Hospitals Seidman Cancer Center and
Cleveland Clinic Taussig Cancer Institute
Cleveland, Ohio
UH Seidman Cancer Center
800.641.2422 • *uhhospitals.org/services/cancer-services*
CC Taussig Cancer Institute
866.223.8100 • *my.clevelandclinic.org/departments/cancer*
Case CCC
216.844.8797 • *case.edu/cancer*

City of Hope National Medical Center
Duarte, California
800.826.4673 • *cityofhope.org*

Dana-Farber/Brigham and Women's Cancer Center |
Mass General Cancer Center
Boston, Massachusetts
877.442.3324 • *youhaveus.org*
617.726.5130 • *massgeneral.org/cancer-center*

Duke Cancer Institute
Durham, North Carolina
888.275.3853 • *dukecancerinstitute.org*

Fox Chase Cancer Center
Philadelphia, Pennsylvania
888.369.2427 • *foxchase.org*

Fred & Pamela Buffett Cancer Center
Omaha, Nebraska
402.559.5600 • *unmc.edu/cancercenter*

Fred Hutchinson Cancer Center
Seattle, Washington
206.667.5000 • *fredhutch.org*

Huntsman Cancer Institute at the University of Utah
Salt Lake City, Utah
800.824.2073 • *healthcare.utah.edu/huntsmancancerinstitute*

Indiana University Melvin and Bren Simon
Comprehensive Cancer Center
Indianapolis, Indiana
888.600.4822 • *www.cancer.iu.edu*

Mayo Clinic Comprehensive Cancer Center
Phoenix/Scottsdale, Arizona
Jacksonville, Florida
Rochester, Minnesota
480.301.8000 • *Arizona*
904.953.0853 • *Florida*
507.538.3270 • *Minnesota*
mayoclinic.org/cancercenter

Memorial Sloan Kettering Cancer Center
New York, New York
800.525.2225 • *mskcc.org*

Moffitt Cancer Center
Tampa, Florida
888.663.3488 • *moffitt.org*

O'Neal Comprehensive Cancer Center at UAB
Birmingham, Alabama
800.822.0933 • *uab.edu/onealcancercenter*

Robert H. Lurie Comprehensive Cancer
Center of Northwestern University
Chicago, Illinois
866.587.4322 • *cancer.northwestern.edu*

Roswell Park Comprehensive Cancer Center
Buffalo, New York
877.275.7724 • *roswellpark.org*

Siteman Cancer Center at Barnes-Jewish Hospital
and Washington University School of Medicine
St. Louis, Missouri
800.600.3606 • *siteman.wustl.edu*

St. Jude Children's Research Hospital/
The University of Tennessee Health Science Center
Memphis, Tennessee
866.278.5833 • *stjude.org*
901.448.5500 • *uthsc.edu*

Stanford Cancer Institute
Stanford, California
877.668.7535 • *cancer.stanford.edu*

The Ohio State University Comprehensive Cancer Center -
James Cancer Hospital and Solove Research Institute
Columbus, Ohio
800.293.5066 • *cancer.osu.edu*

The Sidney Kimmel Comprehensive
Cancer Center at Johns Hopkins
Baltimore, Maryland
410.955.8964
www.hopkinskimmelcancercenter.org

The UChicago Medicine Comprehensive Cancer Center
Chicago, Illinois
773.702.1000 • *uchicagomedicine.org/cancer*

The University of Texas MD Anderson Cancer Center
Houston, Texas
844.269.5922 • *mdanderson.org*

UC Davis Comprehensive Cancer Center
Sacramento, California
916.734.5959 • *800.770.9261*
health.ucdavis.edu/cancer

UC San Diego Moores Cancer Center
La Jolla, California
858.822.6100 • cancer.ucsd.edu

UCLA Jonsson Comprehensive Cancer Center
Los Angeles, California
310.825.5268 • uclahealth.org/cancer

UCSF Helen Diller Family
Comprehensive Cancer Center
San Francisco, California
800.689.8273 • cancer.ucsf.edu

University of Colorado Cancer Center
Aurora, Colorado
720.848.0300 • coloradocancercenter.org

University of Michigan Rogel Cancer Center
Ann Arbor, Michigan
800.865.1125 • rogelcancercenter.org

University of Wisconsin Carbone Cancer Center
Madison, Wisconsin
608.265.1700 • uwhealth.org/cancer

UT Southwestern Simmons
Comprehensive Cancer Center
Dallas, Texas
214.648.3111 • utsouthwestern.edu/simmons

Vanderbilt-Ingram Cancer Center
Nashville, Tennessee
877.936.8422 • vicc.org

Yale Cancer Center/Smilow Cancer Hospital
New Haven, Connecticut
855.4.SMILOW • yalecancercenter.org

Notes

Index

Made in United States
Troutdale, OR
01/21/2025

28192343R00055